GUTBUSTER
RECIPES

Other books by Rosemary Stanton

The diet dilemma
Eating for life
Food for under 5s
Food for health
Food and you
Rosemary Stanton's complete book of food
    and nutrition
The GutBuster waist loss guide
    (with Garry Egger)
Eating for Peak Performance
Rosemary Stanton's healthy cooking
The Good Gut Cookbook
Rosemary Stanton's fat and fibre counter

GUTBUSTER
RECIPES

Rosemary Stanton

Cartoons by Sue Plater

ALLEN & UNWIN

First published 1994
Allen & Unwin Pty Ltd
9 Atchison Street, St Leonards, NSW 2065 Australia

National Library of Australia
Cataloguing-in-Publication entry:

Stanton, Rosemary
  GutBuster recipes.

  Includes index.
  ISBN 186373 703 0.

  1. Low-fat diets—Recipes. 2. Reducing diets—Recipes.
  I. Egger, Garry. The gut buster waist loss guide.
  II. GutBuster recipes. III. Title.

641.5635

Set in 11/14 pt Souvenir by DOCUPRO, Sydney
Printed by Griffin Paperbacks, Adelaide

10 9 8 7 6 5 4 3

Contents

Introduction

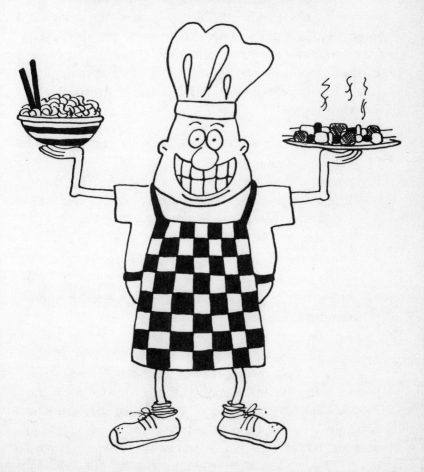

The GutBuster Program is for men who want to lose their paunch, or pot-belly. It is an educational, knowledge-based program designed specifically for men; it therefore differs from the majority of weight loss programs which are designed for women and don't suit the lifestyle and habits of most men.

The GutBuster Program is *not* a diet. Nor is it one of those useless wonder programs that promise you wonderful results for little effort—and don't work for more than a couple of weeks. Instead, the GutBuster Program gives you information about the specific problems of a pot-belly and its health hazards and then gives you a plan for doing something about the problem. This involves:

- changing habits that encourage over-eating and under-exercising
- moving more throughout the day—not by doing sit-ups and exercises that you may not like, but with a program based on working more exercise into your day and walking more
- eating less fat and more fibre, but *not* necessarily eating *less* food
- trading off a limited amount of alcohol for more exercise or fewer fatty foods.

The GutBuster Program started in Newcastle, Australia. It has now spread throughout Australia and is also being set up in many other countries including New Zealand, Canada and the United States. The program involves an introductory course and advanced courses, including a health screening. There is also a

GutBuster Club providing information, a newsletter and more health tests.

To go with the program, Garry Egger and I wrote the *GutBuster Waist Loss Guide*. It's been a great success and thousands of men have found that someone has their interests at heart. Since then, we have been inundated with requests for a recipe book to go with the *GutBuster Waist Loss Guide*. Here it is.

Like the GutBuster Program, this book is aimed at men. If you've always had a secret yearning to cook, here's your chance. The recipes have been designed for people who

- want good-tasting food
- want food that's filling
- want food that's easy to prepare
- don't have much time to cook elaborate meals.

No previous cooking experience is needed and you'll find other people will enjoy the results without having any idea they're eating low-fat foods.

The GutBuster Program emphasises what you *can* have rather than what you *can't*. You won't feel hungry and you won't be confined to eating lettuce and cottage cheese. Instead, it shows you how to eat heartily and healthily with good-tasting, filling foods. It's not a gee-whiz wonder program with dramatic weight loss (almost invariably followed by its return) and it doesn't involve any drugs, herbs, diet pills, heart-stopping exercise or meal replacements. We want you to eat well and healthily and, above all, to enjoy your food.

The GutBuster Program is not aimed at your weight but at your waist. Research has now established that fat around the waist and on the upper body is a health hazard, increasing the risks of coronary heart disease, high blood pressure, diabetes, gall stones, breast cancer in women and, probably, bowel cancer. By contrast, fat on the lower body around the thighs, hips and bottom is not a hazard for any of these common health problems.

Men of all ages tend to accumulate any excess body fat around the waist and on the upper body. So do older women. But while there is a good weight loss program which attracts women (Weight Watchers), it has proved less attractive to men. The GutBuster Program was therefore devised for men, with a lot of input from men themselves. They even chose the name!

The good news which the GutBuster Program tells you about, is that upper body fat is easier to remove than fat on the lower body. However, it does require eating less fat, and exercise also helps. Not a punishing kind of exercise, but simply moving the body more, building back the kind of exercise that our lifestyle once included.

If you want to move more, it's important to provide the body's muscles with plenty of fuel. This comes from the diet in the form of carbohydrates—foods like bread, potatoes, rice, pasta, beans and fruit. These are good filling foods. Unfortunately when some people try to increase their intake of these foods, they inadvertently add lots of fat—thereby negating the benefits. The recipes in this book are therefore low in fat, but not so low that eating becomes a miserable experience. That's not part of the GutBuster Program. Instead, you'll find that you can cook delicious meals *and* keep your fat intake down to appropriate gut buster levels. I have included the fat content of each recipe to make it easy for you to follow the GutBuster philosophy. You don't need to count calories on the GutBuster Program because we know that calories from fats are more fattening than those from carbohydrates.

The GutBuster Program emphasises changing habits without losing the enjoyment of your present lifestyle. To make that easy, I have included healthy low-fat recipes for barbecues. You'll get lots of flavour, plenty of food—but much less fat. If you don't tell your mates they're eating foods with less fat, they'll probably never know. This is not light cooking in the sense of delicate portions: it *is* light in being low in fat.

There are also recipes for healthy high-fibre, low-fat stir-fries (surely one of the quickest and easiest ways to cook) because I know that most people don't have a lot of time to cook. As well, I have included plenty of pasta dishes, great soups, some rice dishes, some new ways with good filling potatoes, and some interesting salads (definitely not just rabbit food). There are even desserts!

Using these recipes will help you to follow the GutBuster Program.

I hope you enjoy cooking and eating your way through!

Rosemary Stanton, 1994

Soups

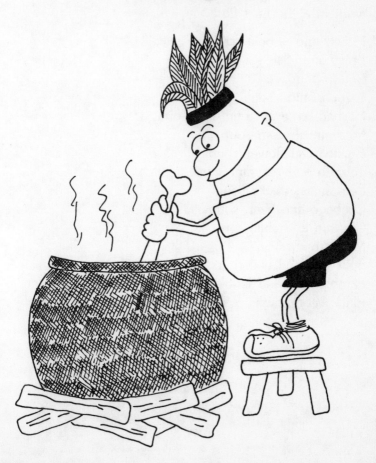

Soups are filling and can be hearty foods. Add some
bread, rolls and fruit, and you have a healthy, low-fat
meal. Or, if you often feel hungry between meals, make
a big pot of soup and help yourself to a ladle or two.
Heat it in the microwave and you have a healthy,
satisfying snack.

All the recipes in this section are low in fat. Some
are ideal winter warmers and can easily be taken to
work in a thermos flask.

Prawn and noodle soup
Spicy sour fish soup
Potato soup
French onion soup
Herbed butternut pumpkin soup
Fresh mushroom soup
Curried cauliflower soup
Tomato and zucchini soup
Peasant vegetable soup
Cabbage and bean soup
Chicken and chilli soup
Minestrone
Split pea and bacon soup
Lamb shank and lentil soup
Black bean soup

Prawn and noodle soup

A hearty meal-in-one-dish soup with loads of flavour.

300 g green prawns
2 teaspoons olive oil
1 large or 2 medium onions, sliced
1 clove garlic
1 teaspoon chopped fresh ginger*
1 teaspoon chopped chilli
1 tablespoon Thai seasoning*
2 cups sliced broccoli
6 cups water
250 g fine rice noodles
½ cup chopped fresh coriander

* available in jars in supermarket or delicatessen

1. Shell and de-vein prawns, leaving tails on.
2. Heat oil in a non-stick pan and cook onion, garlic, ginger, chilli and Thai seasoning over a gentle heat for about 5 minutes. Add broccoli and toss well.
3. Add water and bring to the boil. Cook for about 5 minutes then add prawns and noodles. Continue cooking until noodles are done (about 3 minutes) and prawns are pink. Serve in large soup bowls and sprinkle with coriander.

———————————————————

Serves 4
Fat per serve: 3 grams

Spicy sour fish soup

This soup has a Thai influence in its flavours. Goes well with a Thai meal.

6 cups water
1 fish head or 1 cup prawn shells (save from another dish or ask at your local fish shop)
1 stalk lemon grass, including lower white part*
3 lime or lemon leaves
1 teaspoon chopped fresh chillies
500 g boneless fish fillets, diced
1 cup sliced green shallots
1 red capsicum, seeded and cut into strips
125 g button mushrooms, sliced
2 tablespoons lime juice
1 tablespoon fish sauce
1 cup chopped fresh coriander

* available in jars in supermarket or delicatessen or fresh from the greengrocer

1. Bring water to the boil, add fish head (or prawn shells), lemon grass, lime or lemon leaves. Cover and simmer for 10 minutes. Strain off liquid, reserving it for the soup.
2. Strain stock and add fish, shallots, capsicum, mushrooms, lime juice and fish sauce. Continue cooking until fish is tender. Add coriander. Serve at once.

Serves 4
Fat per serve: 1 to 5 grams,
depending on variety of fish used.

Potato soup

A filling and comforting soup on cold winter days (or nights).

4 cups chicken stock
750 g potatoes, peeled
1 medium leek, washed and sliced
3 bay leaves
1 teaspoon mixed dried herbs
¾ cup skim milk powder
pinch nutmeg
1 tablespoon chopped dill

1. Combine stock, potatoes, leek, bay leaves and herbs in a large saucepan, bring to the boil, cover and simmer for 15 to 20 minutes or until potatoes are tender. Remove bay leaves.
2. Blend soup with skim milk powder and nutmeg until smooth. Return to saucepan, heat, stirring constantly (take care not to let it burn when it splutters). Serve topped with dill.

Serves 4
Fat per serve: 0

French onion soup

If you use a fat-reduced cheddar (7% fat), this soup is fine for gut busters.

    1 kg onions, sliced thinly
    1 tablespoon olive oil
    2 teaspoons sugar
    5 cups beef stock
    ¼ cup dry sherry
    4 bay leaves
    1 teaspoon dried thyme
    4 slices French bread
    4 teaspoons French mustard
    ½ cup (50 g) fat-reduced cheddar cheese, grated

1. Heat oil in a large heavy-based pot, add onion and cook over a very low heat, stirring occasionally, for 30 minutes.
2. Add sugar, stock, sherry, bay leaves and thyme. Bring to the boil, cover and simmer for 10 minutes.
3. While soup is cooking, spread bread with mustard and bake at 180°C for about 5 minutes. Pile cheese onto bread and bake a further 5 to 8 minutes.
4. Place bread into 4 serving bowls. Remove bay leaves, ladle soup over bread and serve at once.

Serves 4
Fat per serve: 7 grams

Herbed butternut pumpkin soup

The hardest part of making pumpkin soup is peeling the pumpkin. Butternuts make it a bit easier.

2 teaspoons olive oil
1 medium onion, chopped
1 kg peeled butternut pumpkin (use about 1.3 kg pumpkin), cut in 3 cm pieces
1 teaspoon dried sage
1 teaspoon dried rosemary
1 teaspoon dried thyme
4 cups chicken stock or water
½ cup low-fat natural yoghurt
1 tablespoon chopped fresh parsley
freshly ground black pepper

1. Heat oil in a large saucepan and gently cook onion for 3 to 4 minutes. Add pumpkin and dried herbs, mix well and stir over moderate heat for 2 to 3 minutes.
2. Add stock, bring to the boil, cover and simmer until pumpkin is soft. Blend until smooth and serve topped with a dollop of yoghurt, a sprinkle of parsley and some pepper.

Serves 4
Fat per serve: 3 grams

Fresh mushroom soup

If you can find or buy field mushrooms, with their rich earthy flavour, this soup is extra good.

2 teaspoons butter
1 medium onion, chopped
1 clove garlic, crushed
500 g mushrooms (preferably dark field mushrooms)
1 teaspoon dried oregano
3 bay leaves
4 cups water
2 tablespoons brandy
2 tablespoons sour light cream
2 tablespoons chopped chives

1. Heat butter in medium saucepan and cook onion and garlic over a gentle heat until softened. Add mushrooms and oregano and continue cooking for a few minutes. Add bay leaves and water, bring to the boil, cover and simmer for about 10 minutes. Remove bay leaves.
2. Blend soup, adding brandy. Return to saucepan and reheat. Pour into bowls, swirl sour light cream through soup and sprinkle with chives.

Serves 4
Fat per serve: 4 grams

Curried cauliflower soup

A spicy Indian-style soup that makes a good start to a meal.

> 1 tablespoon coriander
> 1 teaspoon cumin
> 1 teaspoon turmeric
> 2 teaspoons butter
> 1 medium onion, chopped finely
> 1 teaspoon chopped chilli
> 1 teaspoon chopped fresh ginger
> 1 small cauliflower, sliced
> 4 cups beef or chicken stock
> 1 cup cooked rice
> 2 tablespoons lemon juice

1. Using a non-stick frying pan, cook coriander, cumin and turmeric until they almost begin to burn (do not let them burn).
2. In saucepan, heat butter and cook onion, chilli and fresh ginger over a low heat for 3 to 4 minutes. Scrape spices from pan into onion, add cauliflower and stir well together. Add stock, bring to the boil, cover and simmer until cauliflower is tender. Tip rice into soup, cook a further minute or two until rice is hot. Add lemon juice.

Serves 4
Fat per serve: 2 grams

Tomato and zucchini soup

The flavour of tomatoes and mint is very good. This soup reheats well and can easily be carried in a thermos for lunch.

    1 tablespoon olive oil
    2 large onions, chopped roughly
    2 cloves garlic
    1 packet chicken noodle soup mix
    1 kg zucchini, sliced
    1 kg tomatoes, chopped
    5 cups water
    2 or 3 sprigs fresh mint
    1 teaspoon sugar
    freshly ground pepper
    1 tablespoon chopped mint

1. Heat oil in large saucepan and gently cook onion, garlic and dry soup mix for 4 to 5 minutes. Add zucchini, tomatoes, water, sprigs of mint, sugar and pepper. Bring to the boil, cover and simmer for about 10 minutes, or until zucchini is tender.
2. Puree soup until smooth. Serve topped with chopped mint.

Serves 6
Fat per serve: 4 grams

Peasant vegetable soup

Make a big pot of this soup, have it for a simple lunch or help yourself to a bowl between meals.

6 cups chicken stock
¾ cup red lentils
10 cups chopped vegetables (choose any or all of:
    broccoli, cauliflower, onion, potato, pumpkin,
    zucchini, cabbage, carrot, parsnip, squash,
    mushrooms, spinach, peas, green beans)
½ cup chopped parsley
freshly ground black pepper

Bring chicken stock to the boil, add lentils and cook for 10 minutes. Add vegetables, cover and simmer for about 10 minutes or until vegetables are tender. Serve topped with parsley and pepper.

Serves 4 to 6
Fat per serve: 0

Cabbage and bean soup

This is a thick and hearty soup that serves as a meal. Great on cold days.

    4 slices French bread
    1 clove garlic, peeled and cut in half
    2 teaspoons olive oil
    1 medium onion, chopped finely
    1 clove garlic, crushed
    1 teaspoon dried thyme
    1 medium carrot, sliced
    2 medium zucchini, sliced
    2 cups chicken stock
    400 g can four-bean mix, drained
    400 g can tomatoes, no added salt
    2 cups shredded green cabbage
    1 red capsicum, seeded and sliced

1. Rub bread with cut clove of garlic. Place on oven shelf and bake at 180°C for 15 minutes until crisp.
2. Heat oil and gently cook onion, garlic and thyme for 2 to 3 minutes. Add carrot and zucchini and continue cooking for 1 to 2 minutes.
3. Add stock, beans, tomatoes, cabbage and capsicum, bring to the boil and cook, uncovered, for 10 minutes.
4. Place a slice of the oven-toasted bread into each bowl and ladle soup over the top. Serve at once.

Serves 4
Fat per serve: 3 grams

Chicken and chilli soup

The chicken legs give an excellent flavour. If you don't like too much heat, reduce chilli.

6 skinless chicken legs
4 cups water
1 medium onion, chopped finely
5 or 6 parsley stalks
2 cups shredded cabbage
440 g can corn kernels
400 g can tomatoes
1 cup sliced green shallots
2 small red chillies, seeded and chopped
1 lime

1. Place chicken, water, onion and parsley into a large saucepan. Bring to the boil, cover and simmer for 30 minutes. Remove parsley stalks.
2. Add cabbage, corn (and surrounding liquid), tomatoes and green shallots. Cook, covered, for a further 5 minutes.
3. Place chopped chilli in bowl, ladle soup over the top and squeeze lime juice over.

Serves 4 to 6
Fat per serve: 2 grams

Minestrone

The Italians add some crusty bread and make a meal of this.

6 cups chicken stock
1 cup black-eyed beans
1 large onion, chopped finely
1 stick celery, sliced
2 medium carrots, sliced finely
1 leek, washed and sliced
800 g can tomatoes, chopped roughly
1 teaspoon dried basil
4 bay leaves
100 g small pasta shells
2 cups shredded English spinach
1 cup sliced mushrooms
2 tablespoons chopped parsley
2 tablespoons Parmesan cheese

1. Heat stock and add beans, onion, celery, carrot, leek, tomatoes, basil and bay leaves. Bring to the boil, cover and simmer for 30 minutes.
2. Add pasta, spinach and mushrooms and simmer for another 10 minutes. Remove bay leaves. Serve sprinkled with parsley and cheese.

Serves 6
Fat per serve: 1 gram

Split pea and bacon soup

Make sure you ask the butcher or delicatessen for lean bacon bones.

250 g bacon bones
8 cups water
375 g green split peas
1 medium onion, chopped finely
10 cm piece of celery, sliced finely
3 bay leaves
1 teaspoon dried thyme leaves
2 medium potatoes, diced
1 cup frozen peas
1 tablespoon lemon juice

1. Place bacon bones, water, split peas, onion, celery, bay leaves and thyme in a large saucepan. Bring to the boil, cover and simmer for 45 minutes or until peas are tender. Remove bay leaves and bacon bones.
2. Add potatoes and simmer until tender. Add frozen peas and continue cooking until peas are hot. Serve sprinkled with lemon juice.

Serves 6
Fat per serve: 2 grams

Lamb shank and lentil soup

A meal in itself, this soup is one for days when you're feeling hungry. Long cooking time but you can go off and do something else while the soup is cooking.

2 lamb shanks, trimmed of fat
1 large onion, chopped
2 teaspoons mixed dried herbs
4 bay leaves
6 cups water
1 cup orange juice
1 cup brown lentils
½ cup brown rice
2 carrots, sliced
4 medium zucchini, sliced
250 g frozen peas

1. Heat a large flameproof casserole or saucepan and brown shanks on all sides. Add onion and herbs and cook, covered, stirring occasionally, for 4 to 5 minutes.
2. Add bay leaves, water, orange juice and lentils. Bring to the boil, cover and simmer for 1½ hours.
3. Add rice and carrots, cover and cook for another 20 minutes.
4. Remove shanks and separate meat from bones. Add meat, zucchini and frozen peas and simmer for about 5 minutes.

Serves 6
Fat per serve: 3 or 4 grams,
depending on size of shanks

Black bean soup

A spicy soup that usually appeals to anyone who likes well-flavoured stick-to-your-ribs food. Good to make on weekends. Black beans are available from health food shops or Asian food stores.

400 g black beans
1 medium onion, chopped
1 large carrot, chopped
125 g mushrooms, sliced
1 clove garlic, crushed
2 teaspoons dried oregano
2 tablespoons paprika
1 teaspoon chopped chilli
400 g can tomatoes
6 cups water
½ cup low-fat natural yoghurt
extra chopped chilli (optional)

1. Cover beans with water and soak overnight. Drain.
2. Combine beans, onion, carrot, mushrooms, garlic, oregano, paprika, chilli, tomatoes and water. Bring to the boil, cover and simmer for 2 hours.
3. Puree soup in blender, return to saucepan to reheat. Serve with a swirl of yoghurt and extra chilli (optional).

Serves 6
Fat per serve: 0

Barbecues

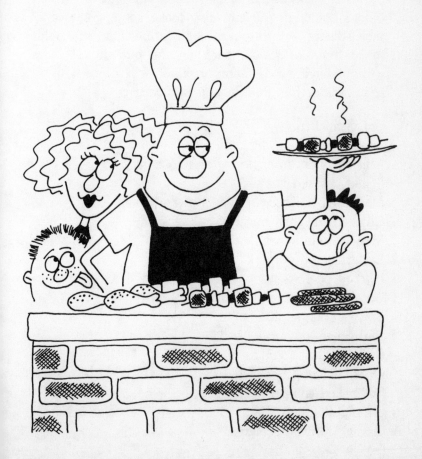

When it comes to barbecues, most men suddenly find
their 'cooking legs'. They can go outside, have a few
beers and socialise while the food is cooking. The meal
is basic, unfussy—and, sadly, fatty. Most Aussie barbecues have become a gut-growing gorging session. It
doesn't have to be like that. You can easily turn on a
gut buster's barbecue.

The secret to fabulous low-fat barbecuing—with lots
of flavour—lies in marinading meat, seafoods or chicken
before cooking. You can also make some great vegetable dishes on the barbecue. Interesting vegetables
make it easier to cut back on the quantity of meat
without having a half-empty plate. Try some of these
easy recipes for great-tasting barbecues.

Spicy chicken
Tangy grapefruit chicken
Chicken with lime, honey and rosemary
Italian chicken kebabs
Marinated mushroom and chicken kebabs
Chicken 'n' chilli burgers
Minted lamb kebabs
Eastern lamb burgers
Herbed beef steaks
Barbecued pork and prune burgers
Spicy coriander fish
Barbecued salmon with dill
Barbecued fish cutlets
Oriental barbecued fish
Foil-baked jewfish
Simply stunning snapper
Orange teriyaki scallops

Barbecued octopus with Italian-style sauce
Honey sesame prawns
Spicy skewered prawns

Spicy chicken

Chicken thighs have an excellent flavour. Without their skin and with any fat trimmed away, they're still moist and delicious. This recipe has loads of flavour.

600 g skinless chicken thighs, trimmed of fat
1 cup natural low-fat yoghurt
2 cloves garlic, crushed
2 tablespoons green curry paste mixture*
    or use a mixture of
    2 tablespoons ground coriander
    1 teaspoon ground cumin
    1 teaspoon turmeric
    1 teaspoon chopped red chilli*
    1 teaspoon chopped fresh ginger*
    1 tablespoon lemon juice

Sauce
1 cup natural low-fat yoghurt
½ cup chopped fresh mint
½ cup chopped fresh coriander
1 tablespoon lime juice

* available in jars

1. Combine yoghurt, garlic, curry paste *or* spice mixture in a shallow bowl. Place chicken thighs into mixture and turn to coat well. Leave in fridge for at least 30 minutes, preferably longer.
2. Cook chicken thighs on barbecue for about 15–20 minutes, turning once and spooning any remaining marinade over chicken.
3. For sauce, combine yoghurt, mint, coriander and lime juice and serve chicken topped with a dollop.
4. Steamed rice or flat bread and a green salad go well.

Serves 4
Fat per serve: 8 grams

Tangy grapefruit chicken

Grapefruit in season are sweet and flavoursome. They make an excellent marinade for chicken. This recipe can also be cooked in a moderate oven.

8 chicken lovely legs (no skin)
2 cloves garlic
1 tablespoon green peppercorns
1 cup grapefruit juice
1 cup chopped parsley
2 tablespoons chopped fresh oregano
1 grapefruit, peeled and segmented

1. Place chicken legs in a shallow dish.
2. Pound together garlic, peppercorns, grapefruit juice, parsley and oregano. Pour over chicken and refrigerate for at least an hour (or overnight).
3. Barbecue chicken legs for about 25–30 minutes, using gentle heat and brushing with marinade several times. Place a grapefruit segment on each chicken leg and leave on barbecue for 1–2 minutes to warm grapefruit.

Serves 4
Fat per serve: 5 grams

Chicken with lime, honey and rosemary

This is one of the simplest ways to cook flavoursome chicken. Use lemon if you can't find lime. By removing any fat and the thick pieces of skin at the neck and rear end, you reduce the fat.

3 small chickens (no. 9)*
finely grated rind and juice of 1 lime
¼ cup finely chopped fresh rosemary
1 tablespoon salt-reduced soy sauce
1 tablespoon honey
2 cloves garlic, crushed

* if you can't find very small chickens, use 1½ larger chickens and use ¼ of a chicken for each person

1. Using kitchen scissors or a sharp knife, split chickens down the centre and flatten out. Remove any visible fat and cut away skin from rear and neck ends of birds. Cut off wing tips.
2. Combine juice, rind, rosemary, soy sauce, honey and garlic. Brush over both sides of chickens, cover and leave in the fridge for at least 12 hours, or up to 24.
3. Grill chickens on barbecue, brushing with marinade mixture and turning several times until cooked. (Cooking times vary. If you have a barbecue with a hood, they take about 25–30 minutes; on a regular barbecue they may take 40–45 minutes.)

Serves 6
Fat per serve: 6–8 grams, depending on how much skin you remove

Italian chicken kebabs

You can arrive home from work and have these ready to eat within 30 minutes.

8 bamboo skewers
600 g skinless chicken breast, cut into cubes
1 cup bottled tomato and eggplant pasta sauce
1 medium eggplant, cut into 3 cm cubes (leave skin on)
1 red or green capsicum, seeded and cut into 3 cm cubes

1. Place skewers in cold water to soak (helps prevent burning).
2. Combine chicken and pasta sauce and leave for 10 minutes.
3. Thread chicken, eggplant and capsicum onto skewers. Barbecue for 10–12 minutes, turning several times and brushing with pasta sauce.
4. Serve with noodles or some type of pasta and a green salad.

Serves 4
Fat per serve: 6 grams

Marinated mushroom and chicken kebabs

The vegetables make this chicken dish more interesting.

8 bamboo skewers
500 g skinless chicken breast fillet, cut into 3 cm
  cubes
2 tablespoons lemon juice
2 tablespoons hoisin sauce*
12 button mushrooms
12 cherry tomatoes
1 red capsicum, seeded and cut into 3 cm cubes
1 green capsicum, seeded and cut into 3 cm cubes

* available from most supermarkets, delicatessens or
  Asian food stores

1. Place skewers in cold water to soak.
2. Combine chicken, lemon juice and hoisin sauce.
   Cover and refrigerate for 30 minutes.
3. Thread chicken, mushrooms, tomatoes and capsicum onto skewers.
4. Barbecue for 10–12 minutes, brushing with remaining marinade and turning several times.

Serves 4
Fat per serve: 5 grams

Chicken 'n' chilli burgers

Chicken burgers are a bit lighter than beef or lamb burgers but they're still delicious and filling. They're also good cold the next day for lunch. Use a food processor to make crumbs, grate vegetables and combine mixture.

3 slices wholemeal bread
400 g minced chicken
1 egg
1 teaspoon chopped fresh chilli
½ cup grated zucchini
½ cup grated carrot
2 tablespoons lemon juice
4 hamburger buns, preferably wholemeal
2 tablespoons fruit chutney
2 medium tomatoes, sliced
8 slices cucumber
4 lettuce leaves

1. Place bread into food processor or blender to make into crumbs. Combine chicken, breadcrumbs, egg, chilli, zucchini, carrot and lemon juice. Form into 4 patties. Barbecue until browned and cooked through, about 10–12 minutes.
2. Split and toast buns. On one half, spread the chutney, top with chicken burger patty, tomatoes, cucumber, lettuce and remaining half bun. Serve at once.

___

Serves 4
Fat per serve: 11 grams

Minted lamb kebabs

There are now wonderful lean cuts of lamb that are tender and full of flavour. Without bones or skin, they are also quick to prepare.

8 bamboo skewers
500 g lean boneless lamb fillet or steaks, cut into
  cubes
½ cup chopped fresh mint
½ cup sliced shallots
½ cup mint jelly (home-made or purchased)
¼ cup red wine
freshly ground pepper

1. Soak some bamboo skewers in cold water (this stops them burning).
2. In a shallow container, combine lamb, mint, shallots, jelly, wine and pepper. Cover and refrigerate for about 20 minutes.
3. Thread meat onto skewers and cook on barbecue, turning and brushing with marinade several times. Do not overcook. Serve with wedges of lemon.

Serves 4
Fat per serve: 6 grams

Eastern lamb burgers

Try these lamb burgers with a difference. The bulgur adds bulk and fibre and makes the lamb go further, cutting down on fat.

1 cup bulgur (cracked wheat)
1 cup boiling water
350 g minced lean lamb
½ cup chopped green shallots
½ cup chopped fresh mint
1 tablespoon ground coriander
¼ cup lemon juice
½ cup low-fat natural yoghurt
1 tablespoon chopped mint
1 tablespoon chopped parsley
4 wholemeal pita breads
1 large tomato, diced
1 cup alfalfa sprouts (optional)

1. Place bulgur in a basin, pour boiling water over, cover and leave for 10 minutes (bulgur will absorb water).
2. Combine bulgur, lamb, shallots, mint, coriander and lemon juice. Make into 4 patties, flatten slightly and barbecue on each side for about 5–8 minutes, or until brown.
3. Combine yoghurt, mint and parsley.
4. Place cooked lamb burgers into pita breads, top with tomato and sprouts and add a dollop of the minted yoghurt. Serve at once.

Serves 4
Fat per serve: 10 grams

Herbed beef steaks

Adding a few herbs gives flavour to any meat. The meat servings are smaller than usual, so have plenty of salads and breads available.

1 tablespoon chopped fresh rosemary
1 tablespoon chopped fresh parsley
1 tablespoon chopped fresh oregano
1 clove garlic, crushed
1 tablespoon Dijon mustard
4 lean steaks, about 120 g each

1. Combine herbs, garlic and mustard. Spread onto both sides of steaks.
2. Barbecue for 5–6 minutes, turning once only and brushing with any remaining herb mixture.
3. Serve with vegetables or salad and potatoes baked in foil.

Serves 4
Fat per serve: 10 grams

Barbecued pork and prune burgers

To get lean minced pork, simply ask your butcher to mince some lean pork for you. Some home food processors are also good for mincing.

500 g lean pork mince
½ cup chopped pitted prunes
1 egg
1 cup cooked brown rice
½ cup chopped green shallots
2 tablespoons mango chutney
1 teaspoon dried sage leaves

Sauce
½ cup dried apricots, cut in halves
1 cup orange juice
1 teaspoon cornflour
2 tablespoons lemon juice

1. Combine pork, prunes, egg, rice, shallots, chutney and sage. Mix well, form into 4 patties and flatten slightly. Barbecue using a medium heat for 6–8 minutes on each side, or until brown but not dry.
2. While patties are cooking, make sauce. Heat orange juice and apricots, cover and simmer for 4–5 minutes.
3. Combine cornflour and lemon juice and add to apricot mixture, stirring constantly until thickened.
4. Serve patties with sauce. Goes well with steamed new potatoes and green vegetable or salad.

Serves 4
Fat per serve: 9 grams

Spicy coriander fish

A simple marinade gives flavour to barbecued fish. The same mixture goes well with prawns.

¾ cup natural low-fat yoghurt
2 tablespoons lime or lemon juice
2 tablespoons freshly chopped coriander
2 cloves garlic, crushed
1 teaspoon ground cumin
2 teaspoons ground coriander
1 teaspoon fresh chopped chilli
4 fish cutlets (blue-eye, kingfish or other)

Combine yoghurt, lime juice, fresh coriander, garlic, cumin, ground coriander and chilli. Place fish in a shallow casserole and pour over spicy yoghurt mixture. Leave to stand for 30 minutes, or longer in fridge. Cook on pre-heated barbecue for about 3–4 minutes on each side, brushing several times with marinade. Serve with lime or lemon wedges.

Serves 4
Fat per serve: 2 grams

Barbecued salmon with dill

When you want a luxury barbecue, you can't beat Tasmanian salmon. Be careful not to overcook it or it will be dry.

4 Tasmanian salmon steaks
2 teaspoons olive oil
2 tablespoons chopped dill

Sauce
½ cup white wine
1 tablespoon chopped shallots
2 tablespoons lemon juice
1 cup low-fat yoghurt
1 tablespoon chopped dill

1. Brush salmon steaks with oil and press dill into both sides of fish. Barbecue for no more than 2–3 minutes on each side (fish cooks quickly and dries out fast if overcooked).
2. For sauce: heat wine, shallots and lemon juice and simmer until reduced by half. Add yoghurt and dill but do not reheat. Serve with salmon steaks.

Serves 4
Fat per serve: 10 grams

Barbecued fish cutlets

This is an easy way to cook any type of fish, adding flavour but no fat.

4 fish cutlets (kingfish, blue-eye, ocean perch, gemfish)
¼ cup no-oil dressing
2 teaspoons finely grated lemon rind
2 tablespoons lemon juice
2 tablespoons chopped fresh herbs (parsley, chives,
    basil, dill)

1. Place fish into a shallow dish. Combine dressing, lemon rind and juice and herbs. Pour over fish, cover and refrigerate for 30 minutes.
2. Barbecue fish until cooked, brushing with marinade. (Do not overcook fish; most cutlets will take only 6–8 minutes.)

Serves 4
*Fat per serve: 2–6 grams, depending
on fish used*

Oriental barbecued fish

A touch of spiciness adds interest to fish. Boneless fish fillets (shark) are excellent cooked this way.

750 g boneless fish fillets
1 clove garlic, crushed
1 teaspoon chopped fresh chilli
2 teaspoons chopped fresh ginger
¼ cup lemon juice
2 tablespoons teriyaki sauce
½ cup chopped fresh coriander

1. Cut fish into 8 pieces and place in a shallow dish. Combine garlic, chilli, ginger, lemon juice, teriyaki sauce and half the coriander. Pour over fish, cover and refrigerate for 30 minutes, turning fish pieces once.
2. Barbecue fish pieces, brushing with marinade and cooking only until barely tender. Sprinkle with remaining coriander when cooked.

Serves 4
Fat per serve: 2 grams

Foil-baked jewfish

A whole barbecued fish always looks stunning. Wrapping fish in foil seals in the flavour and juices, giving a succulent, delicious dish.

>   1 × 2 kg jewfish
>   2 teaspoons light olive oil
>   1 small onion, chopped finely
>   150 g mushrooms, sliced
>   2 slices wholemeal bread, made into crumbs
>   grated rind and juice of 1 lemon
>   2 tablespoons chopped fresh mint
>   freshly ground black pepper

1. Heat oil and gently cook onion for 3–4 minutes. Add mushrooms, cover and continue cooking for 2–3 minutes. Add breadcrumbs, lemon rind and juice, mint and pepper. Stir well.
2. Pack mushroom mixture into the cavity of the fish. Wrap fish in a large piece of non-stick foil. Barbecue for 25–30 minutes or until flesh flakes easily. Serve with wedges of lemon.

Serves 4
Fat per serve: 6 grams

Simply stunning snapper

Nothing could be simpler than this easy recipe.

4 plate-sized snapper
2 lemons
bunch fresh lemon thyme (if unavailable, use dill,
   parsley or a mixture of fresh herbs)

1. Cut 4 pieces of non-stick foil, each large enough
   to envelope one fish.
2. Cut lemons in half and place half a lemon inside
   each fish. Divide lemon thyme into 4 portions and
   place one inside each fish. Wrap up to enclose fish
   in foil.
3. Barbecue for 20–25 minutes, or until fish flakes
   easily with a fork. (Cooking time depends on barbecue; if using a hooded barbecue, cooking time is
   usually shorter.) Partially unwrap foil and serve fish.

Serves 4
Fat per serve: 3 grams

Orange teriyaki scallops

Tasmanian scallops are delicious but delicate. Cook them for only a couple of minutes to keep them tender and moist.

4 long or 8 short bamboo skewers
½ cup orange juice
2 teaspoons finely grated orange rind
2 teaspoons chopped ginger
2 tablespoons teriyaki sauce
6 green shallots, sliced
400 g Tasmanian scallops
16 button mushrooms
½ cup white wine
1 teaspoon cornflour

1. Soak skewers in cold water to prevent burning.
2. Combine orange juice, rind, ginger, teriyaki sauce and shallots. Pour over scallops, cover and leave for 1 hour.
3. Remove scallops from marinade and thread onto skewers with mushrooms. Barbecue over gentle heat, turning several times, until just cooked (about 3–5 minutes).
4. While scallops are cooking, place marinade mixture and wine into a small saucepan. Bring to the boil. Combine cornflour and extra orange juice and add to hot marinade mixture, stirring constantly.

Serves 4
Fat per serve: 1 gram

Barbecued octopus with Italian-style sauce

Baby octopus cook quickly but you need to pre-heat the barbecue grill so that they sizzle and do not stew in their own juices.

500 g baby octopus, cleaned, debeaked and cut in halves
1 clove garlic, crushed
1 cup chopped fresh basil
1 cup red wine
2 large tomatoes, diced
1 capsicum, seeded and diced
2 tablespoons tomato paste
freshly ground pepper

1. To octopus add garlic, basil and ½ cup of red wine. Mix well, cover and leave to stand for 12 hours in the refrigerator.
2. Remove octopus from marinade and barbecue for about 10 minutes or until pink and cooked, turning several times.
3. In a small saucepan, combine any remaining marinade with tomato, capsicum, tomato paste, pepper and remaining half cup of wine. Bring to the boil and cook for about 5 minutes. Serve with octopus.

Serves 4
Fat per serve: 1 gram

Honey sesame prawns

When prawns are cheap, try this delicious barbecue idea. It's so simple that it makes entertaining or cooking for the family trouble free.

1 kg green prawns
2 tablespoons honey
2 teaspoons sesame oil
2 tablespoons hoisin sauce
1 tablespoon salt-reduced soy sauce
1 tablespoon lime juice (or use lemon)
1 tablespoon toasted sesame seeds*

* buy toasted sesame seeds or toast them by stirring in a dry frying pan over a low heat until golden brown

1. Combine honey, oil, hoisin and soy sauces and lime juice. Place unpeeled prawns in this mixture, cover and refrigerate for at least an hour.
2. Cook prawns on barbecue (leave shells on) until they turn red. Serve with toasted sesame seeds to sprinkle on when prawns are peeled.

Serves 4
Fat per serve: 7 grams

Spicy skewered prawns

Another good recipe if you're entertaining. Simple and healthy.

4 long or 8 short bamboo skewers
750 g green prawns
1 clove garlic, crushed
1 teaspoon chopped fresh red chillies
1 tablespoon crushed coriander seeds
1 small onion, chopped finely
2 tablespoons white vinegar
1 tablespoon salt-reduced soy sauce
½ cup tomato puree
1 green capsicum, cut into 2.5 cm pieces
1 red capsicum, cut into 2.5 cm pieces

1. Soak skewers in cold water (to prevent burning).
2. Remove heads and shells from prawns but leave tails on. Place in shallow dish.
3. Combine garlic, chilli, coriander seeds, onion, vinegar, soy sauce and tomato puree. Pour over prawns, cover and refrigerate for several hours.
4. Thread prawns and capsicum onto skewers and barbecue until cooked, brushing with a little of the marinade mixture.
5. Heat any remaining marinade in a small saucepan and serve over cooked prawns. Serve with steamed rice.

Serves 4
Fat per serve: 3 grams

Stir-fries

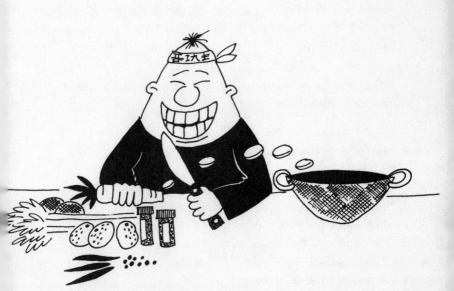

Stir-frying is quick, easy and healthy. There are several ways to do it, using either:

- a wok
- a heavy-based, non-stick frying pan
- a heavy-based, non-stick frying pan brushed with a little oil
- a heavy-based, non-stick frying pan and some concentrated chicken stock
- a non-stick electric frypan

Stir-frying is easy, healthy and particularly suitable for modern lifestyles because it is so fast. Stir-frying also enables you to include lots of vegetables and take meat away from being the centre of the plate to being just one of the ingredients of the meal. This makes a lot of sense from the health point of view. Stir-frying is also ideal because it means you can use up small quantities of a variety of ingredients—which makes it economical as well.

Stir-fried honey chicken
Stir-fried chicken with lemon and spinach
Chicken and greens stir-fry
Chicken with lemon grass and basil
Stir-fried pork and water chestnuts
Stir-fried pork and bean sprouts
Beef and mushroom stir-fry
Chilli beef stir-fry
Stir-fried lamb and fennel
Stir-fried seafoods
Stir-fried squid with basil
Gemfish and rosemary stir-fry

Stir-fried honey chicken

Sweet, but not too sweet, this chicken dish is usually popular with everyone.

2 teaspoons sesame oil
1 large onion, peeled and cut into wedges
400 g skinless chicken stir-fry pieces*
250 g green beans, trimmed
200 g honey snap peas (or use snow peas)
1 red capsicum, seeded and sliced
1 teaspoon chopped fresh ginger
1 tablespoon honey
1 tablespoon salt-reduced soy sauce
1 tablespoon lemon juice
½ cup orange juice

*if stir-fry chicken pieces are not available, use
   chicken breast fillet cut into strips

1. Heat oil in a non-stick pan and cook onion and chicken, turning frequently until chicken is brown (about 6–8 minutes).
2. Add beans, peas, capsicum and ginger and stir-fry for another 3–4 minutes.
3. Combine honey, soy sauce and juices and add to pan. Stir until boiling. Serve at once. Good with steamed rice.

Serves 4
Fat per serve: 8 grams

Stir-fried chicken with lemon and spinach

Try to find the more delicately-flavoured English spinach rather than using silverbeet.

400 g skinless chicken breast fillet, cut into strips
1 teaspoon dried basil leaves
1 bunch English spinach
1 cup sliced green shallots
¾ cup chicken stock
¼ cup lemon juice
2 teaspoons cornflour

1. Using a non-stick pan, cook chicken and basil for 4–5 minutes, or until chicken is brown.
2. Remove stems from spinach and shred leaves. Add to chicken, with shallots and 2 tablespoons of the chicken stock. Stir-fry until spinach begins to soften. Add remaining chicken stock and bring to the boil.
3. Blend lemon juice with cornflour and add, stirring constantly until mixture thickens. Simmer for 1 minute. Serve with rice or cooked couscous.

Serves 4
Fat per serve: 3 grams

Chicken and greens stir-fry

If you're not fond of green vegetables, try them this way and you'll be converted.

2 teaspoons macadamia nut oil
400 g skinless chicken breast strips
1 teaspoon dried oregano
1 cup spring onions or green shallots, cut into 4 cm
   lengths
1 cup sliced broccoli
1 cup sliced green beans
1 cup sliced celery
1 bunch fresh asparagus, cut into 4 cm lengths
1 cup chicken stock
1 cup fresh chopped basil
1 punnet cherry tomatoes

1. Heat oil and stir-fry chicken and oregano for 3–4 minutes.
2. Add spring onions, broccoli, beans, celery and asparagus and cook, tossing ingredients together, for 2–3 minutes.
3. Add chicken stock and bring to the boil. Add basil and cherry tomatoes, stir to combine and serve at once.

Serves 4
Fat per serve: 8 grams

Chicken with lemon grass and basil

If you don't have any fresh lemon grass, it is available in jars.

    2 teaspoons peanut or vegetable oil
    1 tablespoon chopped fresh lemon grass root
    1 clove garlic, crushed
    1 teaspoon chopped chilli
    1 large onion, cut into wedges
    350 g chicken thigh fillets, trimmed of fat
    2 cups sliced green beans
    3 medium tomatoes, cored and cut into wedges
    1 tablespoon fish sauce
    2 tablespoons lemon juice
    1 cup chopped fresh basil

1. Heat oil and gently cook lemon grass, garlic, chilli and onion for 2–3 minutes. Add chicken and stir-fry for 3–4 minutes. Add beans and cook for another 3–4 minutes.
2. Add tomatoes and continue heating until tomatoes are hot but not cooked. Add fish sauce, lemon juice and basil, mix gently and serve at once.

Serves 4
Fat per serve: 9 grams

Stir-fried pork and water chestnuts

Crisp water chestnuts add to this dish. Fresh water chestnuts are available in mid-winter. If using them, boil for about 25 minutes before using.

2 teaspoons oil
1 medium onion, cut into wedges
1 clove garlic, crushed
400 g lean pork steak, cut into strips
2 teaspoons chopped fresh ginger
500 g broccoli, sliced
210 g can water chestnuts, drained and sliced
150 g mushrooms, sliced
1 tablespoon soy sauce
½ cup chicken stock
2 teaspoons cornflour

1. Heat oil and cook onion, garlic and pork for 4–5 minutes, or until pork is brown.
2. Add ginger and broccoli and continue stir-frying for 3–4 minutes. Add water chestnuts and mushrooms and cook for another 2–3 minutes, tossing gently.
3. Combine soy sauce, stock and cornflour. Add to pork and vegetable mixture, stir constantly until mixture boils and thickens. Serve with rice or noodles.

Serves 4
Fat per serve: 9 grams

Stir-fried pork and bean sprouts

This dish can be prepared in about 10 minutes.

    2 teaspoons sesame oil
    400 g lean pork steak, cut into strips
    1 cup sliced green beans
    1 cup sliced green shallots
    2 cups mung bean sprouts
    2 tablespoons oyster sauce
    ½ cup water

1. Heat oil and stir-fry pork for 3–4 minutes.
2. Add beans and shallots and cook for 2–3 minutes.
   Add bean sprouts and toss until hot.
3. Combine oyster sauce and water, add to pork and
   bring to the boil. Serve at once with rice or noodles.

Serves 4
Fat per serve: 9 grams

Beef and mushroom stir-fry

A lighter variation of an old favourite.

2 teaspoons olive oil
1 large onion, sliced
1 clove garlic, crushed
350 g lean rump steak, cut into thin strips
450 g mushrooms, sliced
½ cup red wine
¼ cup tomato paste
¾ cup evaporated skim milk
2 teaspoons cornflour
2 tablespoons chopped fresh parsley

1. Heat oil and stir-fry onion, garlic and steak for 3–4 minutes (do not overcook). Add mushrooms and stir for 2–3 minutes.
2. Combine red wine and tomato paste, add to pan and bring to the boil.
3. Blend milk and cornflour, add to pan and stir constantly until mixture boils and thickens. Sprinkle with parsley. Serve with noodles.

Serves 4
Fat per serve: 8 grams

Chilli beef stir-fry

Hot and spicy, but you can tone it down a bit by reducing the chilli.

2 teaspoons oil
1 large onion, cut into wedges
1 small red chilli, chopped finely
2 tablespoons Mexican spice seasoning*
400 g lean rump or topside steak, cut into strips
1 large red capsicum, seeded and sliced
½ cup water
½ cup chopped fresh parsley

* available in jars

1. Heat oil and stir-fry onion, chilli, Mexican seasoning and steak until meat is lightly browned and tender.
2. Add capsicum and continue cooking for 2–3 minutes. Stir in water and heat to boiling. Serve sprinkled with parsley.

Serves 4
Fat per serve: 9 grams

Stir-fried lamb and fennel

Lean lamb strips are now available and make this dish very easy.

 2 teaspoons olive oil
 2 cloves garlic, crushed
 400 g lamb steaks, cut into strips
 2 teaspoons dried dill
 1 fennel bulb, top removed and sliced
 ½ cup white wine
 1 tablespoon lemon juice
 1 tablespoon fresh chopped dill

1. Heat oil and cook garlic, lamb and dill for 3–4 minutes. Add fennel and continue stir-frying for 2–3 minutes.
2. Combine wine and lemon juice, add to lamb, bring to the boil and simmer for 2 minutes. Sprinkle with fresh dill and serve at once with rice.

Serves 4
Fat per serve: 9 grams

Stir-fried seafoods

You can vary the seafoods according to what looks good at the fish market.

> 1 tablespoon olive oil
> 2 cloves garlic
> 1 large onion, sliced
> 1 teaspoon chopped fresh chilli
> 2 teaspoons chopped fresh ginger
> 500 g fish fillets, cut into chunks
> 350 g green prawns, shelled and deveined (or use
>   scallops or baby octopus)
> 1 cup sliced snow peas
> 1 cup sliced broccoli
> 1 cup chopped fresh coriander

1. Heat oil and cook garlic and onion over a low heat for 3–4 minutes. Add chilli and ginger and cook for a further minute or two. Push to one side of pan.
2. If using octopus, add to pan and cook over a high heat for 3–4 minutes, tossing frequently. Add fish and prawns and stir-fry for about 3 minutes. Remove seafood from pan.
3. Add snow peas and broccoli to pan and stir-fry for 2–3 minutes. Return seafood to pan and stir to combine and heat through. Sprinkle with coriander and serve at once.

Serves 4
Fat per serve: 6 grams

Stir-fried squid with onion and basil

Squid or calamari rings are delicious cooked this way. To prevent them becoming tough, make sure you use a high heat.

3 teaspoons extra virgin olive oil
2 large onions, sliced
2 cloves garlic, crushed
500 g squid hoods
½ cup red wine
2–3 cups fresh basil leaves

1. Using a very low heat and a covered pan, place oil in pan and cook onions and garlic for 45 minutes. Remove onions from pan and set aside.
2. Cut squid into thin rings. Turn heat high under onion pan and cook squid for 2–3 minutes.
3. Return onions to pan and add basil. Toss with squid until heated through. Add red wine, bring to the boil, simmer 1 minute and serve.

Serves 4
Fat per serve: 5 grams

Gemfish and rosemary stir-fry

Substitute any white-fleshed fish for gemfish.

    1 tablespoon olive oil
    1 medium onion, finely chopped
    1 tablespoon chopped fresh rosemary
    1 medium eggplant, cut into strips
    1 medium carrot, cut into thin strips
    500 g gemfish fillets, cut into strips
    1 bunch asparagus, cut into 4 cm lengths
    1 red capsicum, seeded and sliced
    1 green capsicum, seeded and sliced
    ½ cup white wine
    2 tablespoons lemon juice

1. Heat oil and cook onion, rosemary, eggplant and carrot for 3–4 minutes.
2. Add fish, asparagus and capsicums and cook until fish flesh begins to flake.
3. Add wine and lemon juice, bring to the boil and cook for 2 minutes. Serve at once.

Serves 4
Fat per serve: 10 grams (for most other white fish, fat would be 5 grams)

Pasta and rice dishes

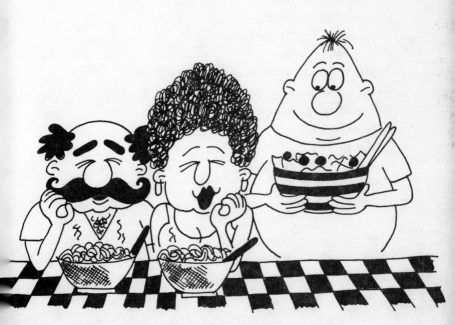

Pasta and rice are both low in fat and high in important complex carbohydrates. Nutritionists recommend them. Unfortunately, many people destroy the nutritional value of pasta by drowning it in fatty sauces. Some also assume that rice must be fried. It doesn't have to be that way. Many delicious pasta and rice dishes are low in fat and high in flavour. Try these and you'll get the idea.

Spaghetti with olives and tomatoes
Red pepper pasta
Fettuccine with spinach and pine nuts
Spaghetti with eggplant and zucchini
Spaghetti Bolognaise
Macaroni with tuna
Pasta with broccoli and chilli
Warm pasta salad
Fettuccine with mushrooms and red wine
Pasta with spinach and ricotta
Rice-stuffed eggplant
Seafood paella
Leeks and rice
Rice and salmon casserole
Corn and rice pie

Spaghetti with olives and tomatoes

This is a simple dish you can have ready in less than 30 minutes.

6 medium tomatoes
500 g spaghetti
1 tablespoon olive oil
1 medium onion, cut into wedges
2 cloves garlic, crushed
½ cup chopped fresh basil (or use parsley)
100 g black olives

1. Cut cores out of tomatoes, place in a bowl and cover with boiling water. Leave to stand for 3–4 minutes, lift tomatoes out of water and remove skins. Cut each tomato into 8 wedges.
2. Cook spaghetti according to packet directions, making sure you don't overcook it.
3. While spaghetti is cooking, heat oil and gently cook onion and garlic over a low heat, stirring occasionally, for 4–5 minutes. Add tomatoes, basil and olives and heat through.
4. Drain spaghetti, place into serving bowls and top with tomato mixture. Serve with a green salad.

Serves 4–5
Fat per serve: 7 grams

Red pepper pasta

Using evaporated skim milk is not the same as using cream, but it still tastes pretty good.

> 400 g pasta (shells, twists or any small, shaped pasta)
> 2 teaspoons olive oil
> 1 large red capsicum, seeded and sliced finely
> 1 medium onion, chopped finely
> 1 teaspoon dried oregano
> freshly ground pepper
> 1 cup evaporated skim milk
> 2 eggs
> 2 tablespoons chopped parsley

1. Cook pasta according to packet directions, taking care not to overcook it. Drain when cooked.
2. While pasta is cooking, heat oil and cook capsicum, onion and oregano, covered, over a gentle heat, stirring occasionally, for 5 minutes.
3. Add drained pasta to capsicum. Season generously with black pepper.
4. Beat milk and eggs and pour into pasta mixture. Cook over a gentle heat, stirring constantly, until mixture boils and thickens. Serve sprinkled with parsley.

Serves 4
Fat per serve: 5 grams

Fettuccine with spinach and pine nuts

If you can find some English spinach rather than silverbeet, the flavour is better.

2 tablespoons pine nuts
400 g spinach fettuccine
2 teaspoons olive oil
1 medium onion, sliced finely
2 cloves garlic, crushed
1 teaspoon dried thyme
1 bunch English spinach
1 tablespoon grated Parmesan cheese

1. Toast pine nuts in a dry frying pan over a low heat, shaking often until golden brown. Do not allow to burn. Set aside.
2. Cook fettuccine according to packet directions, taking care not to overcook.
3. Heat oil in a non-stick frying pan and cook onion, garlic and thyme for 3–4 minutes, stirring often so that onion softens but does not brown too much.
4. Trim stalks from spinach and shred leaves. Add to pan, cover and cook for a few minutes until spinach wilts.
5. Drain fettuccine and serve topped with spinach. Sprinkle each serve with pine nuts and cheese.

Serves 4
Fat per serve: 8 grams

Spaghetti with eggplant and zucchini

If you're short of time, you can skip salting the eggplant and zucchini, but if you can find the time, the eggplant, in particular, has a much better flavour.

1 eggplant, about 600 g, sliced
3 or 4 zucchini, about 400 g, sliced
400 g spaghetti
2 tablespoons no-oil dressing
½ cup chicken stock
½ cup chopped fresh basil

1. Sprinkle eggplant and zucchini with salt. Leave in a colander for about 20 minutes. Rinse under cold water, drain and dry on kitchen paper.
2. Taking batches, grill eggplant and zucchini until soft and beginning to brown on both sides.
3. Cook spaghetti according to directions on packet, taking care not to overcook.
4. Place no-oil dressing and stock in a large pan. Add grilled vegetables and basil and heat through. Serve on top of drained spaghetti.

Serves 4
Fat per serve: 0

Spaghetti Bolognaise

Ever-popular, you can turn spaghetti bolognaise into a gut-buster dish by using very lean mince (look for 95% fat free meat).

400 g spaghetti
400 g lean mince
1 medium onion, chopped finely
1 clove garlic, crushed
1 teaspoon dried basil
400 g can tomatoes, chopped
1 large carrot, grated
250 g mushrooms, sliced
½ cup tomato paste
½ cup red wine

1. Using a heavy-based non-stick pan, cook mince, onion, garlic and basil, stirring occasionally, until meat browns.
2. Add tomatoes, carrot, mushrooms, tomato paste and wine. Bring to the boil and simmer for 30 minutes, stirring occasionally.
3. When sauce has been simmering for about 15 minutes, cook spaghetti according to directions on packet. Drain well. Serve spaghetti topped with bolognaise sauce.

Serves 4
Fat per serve: 5 grams

Macaroni with tuna

This is a meal to make on those occasions when you haven't had time to go shopping. The ingredients for this one are probably in your kitchen cupboard.

400 g macaroni
1 tablespoon olive oil
1 medium onion, chopped finely
1 teaspoon dried mixed herbs
1 diced capsicum *or* 1 cup sliced celery *or* 1 cup sliced mushrooms
400 g can tomatoes, no added salt
400 g can tuna in brine, drained
200 g natural low-fat yoghurt
2 slices wholemeal bread
2 tablespoons grated Parmesan cheese
2 tablespoons chopped fresh parsley

1. Cook macaroni according to directions on packet. Drain.
2. While macaroni is cooking, heat oil and cook onion and herbs over a gentle heat for 3–4 minutes. Add capsicum (or other vegetable) and continue cooking for another 2–3 minutes, stirring several times.
3. Add tomatoes and tuna and heat until boiling.
4. Combine macaroni and yoghurt.
5. Place half the tomato mixture in a greased casserole dish, top with the macaroni mixture and remaining tomato mixture.
6. Process bread into crumbs in food processor or blender. Add cheese and parsley to crumbs and sprinkle over macaroni. Bake in a moderate oven (180°C) for 15 minutes or until crumbs are golden.

Serves 4
Fat per serve: 10 grams

Pasta with broccoli and chilli

With dishes like this, you soon find meatless eating is easy.

500 g pasta (use spaghetti or fettuccine or other
  pasta)
1 tablespoon olive oil
1 medium onion, sliced
2 cloves garlic, crushed
2 teaspoons chilli (or less, if you don't like it hot)
500 g broccoli, sliced
¾ cup chicken stock

1. Cook pasta according to directions on packet, taking care not to overcook.
2. Heat oil in a large heavy-based pan and gently cook onion and garlic for 3–4 minutes. Add chilli and broccoli, cover and cook for 8–10 minutes, stirring often. Add chicken stock and stir well.
3. Serve pasta in bowls and top with broccoli mixture.

Serves 4
Fat per serve: 5 grams

Warm pasta salad

A great salad to serve on its own or with a barbecue.

250 g pasta (twists or shells)
1 cup sliced celery
1 cup diced capsicum (red, green or yellow)
150 g sliced button mushrooms

Dressing
½ cup low-fat yoghurt
1 teaspoon paprika
1 teaspoon grainy mustard
1 tablespoon chopped parsley
1 tablespoon chopped chives
1 tablespoon lemon juice

1. Cook pasta according to directions on packet. Drain well.
2. While pasta is cooking, combine dressing ingredients. Toss through hot pasta. Add celery, capsicums and mushrooms. Serve warm.

Serves 4
Fat per serve: 0

Fettuccine with mushrooms and red wine

Another quick easy dish. The alcohol in wine evaporates during cooking but leaves its wonderful flavour.

500 g fettuccine
1 tablespoon olive oil
1 large onion (preferably a purple onion), sliced finely
2 cloves garlic, crushed
400 g mushrooms, sliced
1 cup red wine
2 tablespoons tomato paste

1. Cook fettuccine according to directions on packet, taking care not to overcook. Drain.
2. While fettuccine is cooking, heat oil in a large heavy-based pan and gently cook onion and garlic for 3 to 4 minutes. Add mushrooms and toss well, cooking for a few minutes until mushrooms begin to soften slightly.
3. Add wine and tomato paste, bring to the boil and boil hard for a minute or two to reduce the volume of the sauce. Pour over fettuccine and serve.

Serves 4–5
Fat per serve: 5 grams

Pasta with spinach and ricotta

A creamy-tasting dish in spite of its low fat content. Use a smooth ricotta for the best texture. If you don't have access to fresh pasta, substitute 500 g dried pasta.

375 g fresh herb and garlic tagliatelle
250 g frozen spinach
250 g low-fat smooth ricotta
1 clove garlic, crushed
¼ cup lemon juice
¼ cup fresh mint sprigs
2 tablespoons fresh marjoram (or use 1 teaspoon dried)
plenty of freshly ground black pepper

1. Cook pasta according to directions on the packet. If using fresh pasta which takes only 2 to 3 minutes cooking, prepare sauce first.
2. Thaw spinach (a microwave makes it fast) and heat in a non-stick pan (or in microwave), stirring until hot.
3. Combine ricotta, garlic, lemon juice, mint and marjoram and blend until smooth. Add spinach. If sauce is too thick, add about ½ cup of the cooking water from the pasta. Toss ricotta/spinach mixture through hot cooked drained pasta.

Serves 4
Fat per serve: 5 grams

Rice-stuffed eggplant

You can vary this dish and use the stuffing in baby pumpkins or capsicums.

½ cup brown rice (or use white or brown/wild rice
   mixture)
⅔ cup water
2 medium eggplants
1 tablespoon olive oil, preferably extra virgin
1 small onion, chopped finely
1 capsicum, preferably red, seeded and diced
½ cup sultanas
1 teaspoon cinnamon
½ teaspoon allspice
¼ teaspoon black pepper
1 cup low-fat cottage cheese
2 tablespoons chopped parsley

1. Combine rice and water in a saucepan with a tightly-fitting lid. Bring to the boil, cover and simmer over a low heat for 20 minutes. All the water will be absorbed.
2. Pierce eggplants with a skewer in several places and bake in a moderate oven for 20 minutes. Remove from oven, cut in half, and when eggplant halves are cool enough to handle, scoop out flesh, leaving enough of a shell to hold the filling. Chop flesh finely.
3. In a small saucepan, heat oil, add onion, cover and cook over a gentle heat, stirring several times, for about 10 minutes. Add capsicum, sultanas, cinnamon, allspice and pepper and continue cooking for another 2 to 3 minutes.

4. Combine cooked rice, eggplant flesh, onion mixture and cottage cheese and mix well. Spoon into capsicum shells, place on a greased dish (preferably the right size to hold the eggplants close together) and bake in a moderate oven for 20 minutes. Sprinkle with chopped parsley and serve.

Serves 4
Fat per serve: 7 grams

Seafood paella

This is an impressive-looking dish and it smells wonderful when cooking. Try to get some saffron threads for their superb flavour. Powdered saffron is not as good.

1 tablespoon olive oil
1 large onion, sliced
1 large red capsicum, seeded and sliced into strips
2 cloves garlic, crushed
1 teaspoon chopped fresh chilli
250 g long grain rice
½ teaspoon coarsely ground black pepper
2 cups chicken stock
1 teaspoon saffron threads (or use ½ teaspoon powdered saffron)
1 cup water
16 mussels, scrubbed
1 tablespoon fresh rosemary leaves, chopped finely
250 g frozen peas
16 prawns (leave shells and heads on)
8 black olives
2 tablespoons lemon juice

1. In a large heavy-based frying pan, heat oil and saute onion, capsicum, garlic and chilli, stirring often, until onion softens.
2. Add rice and pepper and stir well.
3. Heat chicken stock, add saffron.
4. In a large steamer, heat water and steam mussels for 4 to 5 minutes, or until shells open. Discard any that do not open. Strain water and reserve.
5. Add to rice the chicken stock, reserved water from mussels and rosemary. Bring to the boil, turn heat low, cover and simmer for 10 minutes.

6. Add peas and prawns, cover and continue cooking for another 5 to 8 minutes. Decorate with mussels and olives and sprinkle with lemon juice. Serve straight from the pan.

Serves 4
Fat per serve: 7 grams

Leeks and rice

A simple dish to eat with a salad of sliced tomatoes or with barbecued fish.

1 tablespoon olive oil
2 leeks
2 cloves garlic
1 teaspoon dried oregano
2 cups (320 g) fragrant rice
3 cups chicken stock
½ cup white wine

1. Remove tough outer stems from leeks, but reserve green inner core of stem, as well as white parts. Wash well and slice leeks into round pieces.
2. In a large pan (one that has a tight-fitting lid), heat oil and gently cook leeks, garlic and oregano over low to moderate heat until leeks soften. Push to one side of pan.
3. Add rice and stir well for several minutes. Stir rice and leeks together, add stock and wine, bring to the boil, cover, turn heat low and simmer for 15 to 20 minutes (all the liquid should be absorbed).

Serves 4
Fat per serve: 6 grams

Rice and salmon casserole

This is a quick and easy dish to make when you feel like something simple.

1 cup brown rice
1¾ cups water
1 teaspoon dried thyme leaves
400 g can red or pink salmon, drained and flaked
1 red capsicum, seeded and diced
1 cup sliced green shallots
250 g frozen green beans, thawed
2 eggs, beaten
200 g low-fat natural yoghurt
1 teaspoon paprika

1. Place rice, water and thyme in saucepan, bring to the boil, cover and simmer over a low heat for 30 minutes (all the water should be absorbed).
2. Combine rice with remaining ingredients, except paprika. Place in a greased casserole dish, sprinkle with paprika and bake in a moderate oven for 20 minutes.

Serves 4
Fat per serve: 8 grams

Corn and rice pie

A simple dish where you combine everything and pop it into the oven, this is a good way to use up left-over rice and turkey (or chicken).

3 cups cooked rice
1 cup cooked diced turkey (or chicken)
400 g can corn kernels, drained
½ cup sliced green shallots
½ cup sliced celery
1 cup sliced mushrooms
½ red capsicum, seeded and diced
½ green capsicum, seeded and diced
2 tablespoons chopped mint
2 eggs
1 cup evaporated skim milk
1 tablespoon grated Parmesan cheese

1. Combine rice, turkey (or chicken), corn, shallots, celery, mushrooms, capsicum and mint.
2. In blender combine eggs and milk. Pour over rice mixture and mix well. Place into a greased casserole dish, sprinkle with cheese and bake in a moderate oven for 40 minutes.

Serves 4
Fat per serve: 6 grams

Salads

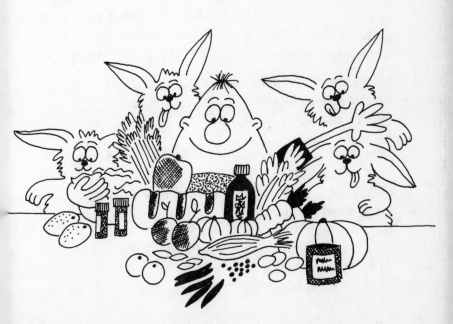

Salads can be crisp and cool and rather flimsy affairs
or they can have some substance with their freshness.
Some are so drowned in dressing that they are no
longer the healthy foods we assume they should be.

These recipes use wonderfully-flavoured salad ingredients with dressings that add tang and interest—with
minimum fat. They are all a far cry from rabbit food.
Some are good to take to work for lunch; others are
best eaten soon after being made. Check the descrip-
tion at the top of each recipe to know which category
each salad fits.

If you have high cholesterol, salad vegetables are
wonderful because they supply a range of antioxidants
which can help prevent the bad form of cholesterol forming
plaque in the arteries. But you don't need to think of such
things when eating—simply enjoy your salads instead.

Italian bread and tomato salad
Potato and lentil salad
Minted chick pea salad
Eggplant salad
Bean salad
Thai chicken salad
Green bean salad with avocado dressing
Pasta salad
Beetroot and horseradish salad
Green salad with egg dressing and crisp croutons
Crunchy pea salad
Mushroom salad
Greek salad
Apple coleslaw
Braised leek salad

Italian bread and tomato salad

This is a hearty salad that tastes best eaten soon after you make it. It goes well with barbecued chicken, fish or lean meat.

4 bread rolls or about 125 g of unsliced bread,
   preferably wholemeal
500 g ripe tomatoes, cut into chunks
1 clove garlic, crushed
1 small onion, peeled and diced
½ cup fresh chopped parsley
1 tablespoon extra virgin olive oil
freshly ground black pepper

1. Cut bread into slices about twice the thickness of regular sliced bread. Place bread on the oven shelf in a moderate oven (180°C) for about 15 minutes, or until it browns and turns crisp. Break into chunks about 1.5 cm square.
2. Combine bread with remaining ingredients. Toss well and eat at once.

Serves 4
Fat per serve: 6 grams

Potato and lentil salad

Nothing even vaguely resembling rabbit food about this salad. Take it to work and enjoy it with a fresh bread roll or some pita bread.

> ¾ cup red lentils
> 2 cups water
> 3 medium–large potatoes (about 450 g), scrubbed
> ½ cup frozen peas
> 1 red capsicum, seeded and diced
> ½ cup sliced celery
> ½ cup chopped Italian parsley
> 2 tablespoons balsamic vinegar (or red wine vinegar)
> 1 tablespoon extra virgin olive oil

1. Place lentils in a saucepan with water, bring to the boil, turn heat low, cover and simmer for 15–20 minutes. Do not allow lentils to cook to a mushy consistency.
2. Microwave or steam potatoes, and dice.
3. Combine cooked lentils, potatoes, frozen peas (the heat of the potatoes will thaw them), capsicum and celery. Leave until cool.
4. Add parsley, vinegar and oil and toss the mixture together. Serve at once or place in fridge until needed.

Serves 4
Fat per serve: 5 grams

Minted chick pea salad

Chick peas have a delightful nutty flavour, are filling and have almost no fat. This hearty salad is excellent to take to work for lunch.

2 × 310 g cans chick peas, drained (or use 2 cups cooked chick peas)
3 medium tomatoes, cored and cut into eight wedges
2 Lebanese cucumbers, diced
½ cup sliced green shallots
1 cup sliced mushrooms
½ cup chopped mint
2 tablespoons lemon juice
1 tablespoon olive or macadamia nut oil
freshly ground black pepper

Combine all ingredients and refrigerate for at least 30 minutes to allow flavours to mingle.

Serves 4
Fat per serve: 5 grams

Eggplant salad

It takes a bit longer to salt and rinse eggplant but the process gets rid of some bitter substances and leaves you with a creamy-flavoured food that makes the effort worthwhile. This salad will last a couple of days in the fridge so it's ideal to take for lunch. It's also delicious with barbecued lean lamb fillets. Make sure you slice the zucchini finely and it won't need cooking.

1 eggplant, about 500 g, sliced
250 g zucchini, sliced finely
1 red capsicum, seeded and sliced
¼ cup red wine
1 tablespoon red wine vinegar
1½ cups pasta sauce (use a bottled variety)
½ cup chopped fresh basil

1. Sprinkle salt over eggplant and zucchini slices and leave for about 20–30 minutes. Rinse salt off and pat vegetables dry using paper towels.
2. Cook eggplant under griller until brown, turn and brown other side.
3. Combine eggplant, zucchini (doesn't need cooking) and capsicum.
4. Mix together wine, vinegar and pasta sauce. Toss through eggplant mixture and sprinkle with basil.

Serves 4
Fat per serve: 0

Bean salad

Bean salads are popular and can easily be taken to work. The flavour usually improves after a few hours. In hot weather, always keep bean dishes in the fridge as these nutritious little morsels are notorious for going 'off'.

310 g can kidney beans, drained
310 g can Lima beans, drained
310 g can chick peas, drained
½ cup sliced green shallots or spring onions
½ cup chopped parsley
2 tablespoons chopped chives
freshly ground pepper
2 Lebanese cucumbers, diced
1 punnet cherry tomatoes, halved
1 tablespoon extra virgin olive oil
1 tablespoon lemon juice

1. Combine beans, chick peas, shallots, parsley, chives, pepper, cucumber and tomatoes. Toss together.
2. Add olive oil and lemon juice and stir gently to combine.

Serves 4
Fat per serve: 5 grams

Thai chicken salad

A more delicate flavour but delicious and guaranteed to tempt the tastebuds.

2 tablespoons lime juice
1 tablespoon soy sauce
½ cup chopped fresh coriander
4 skinless chicken breasts, each cut into 4 pieces
2 teaspoons sesame oil
8 crisp lettuce leaves
12 green shallots, sliced
1 medium carrot, cut into fine strips
1 medium white radish, peeled and cut into fine strips
1 red capsicum, seeded and sliced finely

Dressing
¼ cup rice wine vinegar*
1 teaspoon sugar
1 tablespoon toasted sesame seeds*
½ cup chopped fresh coriander
½ cup chopped fresh basil
2 tablespoons chopped Vietnamese mint**

* available from Asian food stores
** available from Asian greengrocers

1. Combine lime juice, soy sauce and coriander. Add chicken and leave for 30 minutes.
2. Remove pieces of chicken breast from marinade. Heat sesame oil and stir-fry chicken for 3–4 minutes, or until just cooked.
3. Arrange salad vegetables on individual plates. Top with chicken.
4. For dressing, combine vinegar, sugar, sesame seeds and herbs. Combine well and spoon over vegetables.

Serves 4
Fat per serve: 8 grams

Green bean salad with avocado dressing

This is an easy recipe that goes well with barbecued chicken or fish.

500 g green beans, trimmed
1 red capsicum, seeded and sliced

Dressing
½ a ripe avocado
2 teaspoons French mustard
100 g ricotta cheese
100 g low-fat natural yoghurt
2 tablespoons lemon juice

1. Steam or microwave beans until they are just tender. Do not overcook. Immediately tip beans into a colander and hold under the cold tap to stop the cooking and keep beans crisp and green. Drain well.
2. Place avocado, mustard, ricotta, yoghurt and lemon juice into blender and process until smooth.
3. Arrange beans and capsicum on shallow dish and top with dressing.

Serves 4
Fat per serve: 7 grams

Pasta salad

Even people who are not fond of salads usually like pasta salad.

250 g spiral pasta
250 g broccoli tops
2 stalks celery, sliced
1 red capsicum, seeded and diced
1 green capsicum, seeded and diced
1 punnet cherry tomatoes

Dressing
200 g low-fat natural yoghurt
2 tablespoons lemon juice
1 tablespoon chopped chives
½ cup chopped fresh coriander (or use parsley)
2 teaspoons paprika
1 tablespoon grainy mustard

1. Cook pasta according to directions on packet. Drain well.
2. Steam broccoli for 2 to 3 minutes or microwave for 1 to 2 minutes. Immediately tip into a colander and hold under tap to cool and stop cooking. Drain.
3. In a salad bowl combine pasta, broccoli, celery, capsicums and tomatoes.
4. For dressing: combine yoghurt, lemon juice, chives, coriander, paprika and mustard. Pour over pasta and mix well.

Serves 4 to 6
Fat per serve: 0

Beetroot and horseradish salad

Easy to make and with a real bite to it. Excellent with a lean grilled steak. A food processor makes the grating task easier.

    1 bunch fresh beetroot
    2 to 3 teaspoons horseradish (or use 1 tablespoon
        prepared creamed horseradish)
    2 tablespoons wine vinegar
    plenty of freshly ground black pepper

1. Peel beetroot (wear rubber gloves if you don't want stained hands). Remove tops and root. Grate coarsely.
2. Combine beetroot with horseradish, vinegar and pepper. Stand for at least 15 minutes to allow flavours to blend.

Serves 4
Fat per serve: 0

Green salad with egg dressing and crisp croutons

A slightly fancy salad, great if you're entertaining. Goes well with barbecued fish and steamed new potatoes.

3 slices bread, crusts removed
2 teaspoons olive oil
salad bowl of mixed lettuce leaves (use iceberg, oak-leaf, butter, radicchio or any other lettuces available)*

Dressing
2 tablespoons lemon juice
2 tablespoons white wine vinegar
2 teaspoons mustard
1 egg
freshly ground pepper

* some greengrocers sell mixed salad leaves by weight.

1. Heat oil (in a cup in the microwave for 20 seconds is easy). Using a pastry brush, brush it over the bread. Bake bread in a moderate oven for about 20 minutes, or until crisp and brown.
2. Arrange salad leaves in salad bowl.
3. Make dressing by heating lemon juice, vinegar and mustard in a small saucepan (or use a bowl in microwave and heat on High for 30 seconds). Beat egg in a small bowl and pour on the hot lemon mixture. Pour into a small saucepan and stir over a very low heat until it is almost boiling. Do not boil or dressing will curdle. Add pepper to dressing and pour over salad leaves. Toss well and serve at once.

Serves 4
Fat per serve: 4 grams

Crunchy pea salad

Use ingredients from your freezer and pantry as the basis for this salad.

2 cups frozen minted peas
170 g can water chestnuts, drained and sliced
1 red capsicum, seeded and diced
½ cup low-fat natural yoghurt
2 teaspoons Dijon mustard
1 teaspoon dried dill
plenty of freshly ground black pepper

1. Place peas in a strainer and hold under the hot tap until they are just thawed. Drain.
2. Combine peas, water chestnuts and capsicum. Toss with yoghurt, mustard, dill and pepper.

Serves 4
Fat per serve: 0

Mushroom salad

Make this salad at least 30 minutes before you want to eat so the mushrooms can absorb some of the flavours.

2 tablespoons lemon juice
1 tablespoon olive oil
2 tablespoons balsamic vinegar (or use wine vinegar)
1 tablespoon grainy mustard
freshly ground pepper
400 g button mushrooms, sliced
2 tablespoons chopped chives
about 10 green shallots, sliced

1. Combine lemon juice, oil, vinegar, mustard and pepper.
2. Place mushrooms into a bowl, pour over lemon mixture and toss lightly but thoroughly. Top with chives and shallots, cover with plastic wrap and refrigerate for at least 30 minutes. Mix shallots into mushrooms.

Serves 4
Fat per serve: 5 grams

Greek salad

Low-fat fetta cheese is available from many delicatessens and some supermarkets. It crumbles well and even the small quantity in this salad adds loads of flavour.

3 medium-sized tomatoes, cored and diced
3 Lebanese cucumbers, cut into chunks
1 small purple onion, sliced
about half an iceberg lettuce, torn
½ cup parsley sprigs
½ cup crumbled fetta cheese
2 tablespoons low kilojoule dressing
1 tablespoon lemon juice
½ cup (75 g) black olives

1. Combine tomatoes, cucumbers, onion, lettuce and parsley sprigs in a salad bowl. Top with cheese.
2. Sprinkle salad with dressing and lemon juice and toss well. Top with olives.

Serves 4
Fat per serve: 4 grams

Apple coleslaw

Adding some apple to coleslaw sweetens it. Use a food processor for fast slicing.

>   2 red-skinned apples, quartered, cored and cut into
>   thin slices
>   3 tablespoons lemon juice
>   4 cups shredded cabbage
>   1 green capsicum, seeded and sliced
>   2 teaspoons fennel seeds
>   200 g low-fat natural yoghurt
>   ½ cup chopped mint

1. Toss apple slices with lemon juice. Add cabbage, capsicum and fennel seeds and mix gently together.
2. Combine yoghurt and mint and pour over cabbage. Toss well.

Serves 4
Fat per serve: 0

Braised leek salad

*Mediterranean people like salads made from cooked veg-
etables. This one certainly goes well with barbecued
chicken or a strongly-flavoured baked fish.*

2 large or 4 small leeks
1 tablespoon extra virgin olive oil
2 cloves garlic, crushed
1 cup white wine
10 peppercorns
2 bay leaves
1 teaspoon dried rosemary leaves
2 teaspoons finely grated lemon rind
1 tablespoon lemon juice

1. Trim top tough parts of leeks, but do not trim off
   all the green section. If leeks are large, cut in half
   lengthwise. Wash leeks thoroughly, opening green
   leaves with your fingers to remove any lingering
   dirt.
2. Heat oil, add garlic and cook for 1 minute. Add
   leeks, wine, peppercorns, bay leaves, rosemary and
   lemon rind. Simmer, covered, for about 15 to 20
   minutes. Remove bay leaves.
3. Place leeks into a shallow serving dish, add lemon
   juice to cooking pan and pour over leeks. Refrigerate for an hour or longer.

Serves 4
Fat per serve: 5 grams

Potatoes and vegetables

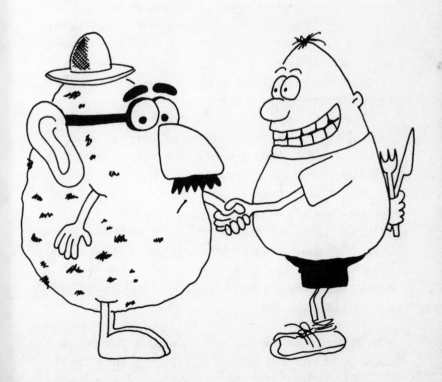

The GutBuster Program has no restrictions on potatoes or other vegetables, but it does restrict fat. That means you need something other than butter, margarine or sour cream to give your spuds and vegies more flavour.

You probably already know that vegetables are good for you. They're full of vitamins, for a start. But vitamins are just one part of the long line-up of nutritional goodies in vegetables. They also have plenty of fibre which helps prevent constipation and many minerals that are needed by muscles and blood.

The latest 'wonder' ingredients in vegetables are antioxidants. Brightly-coloured vegetables contain literally hundreds of these substances that help prevent damage to arteries and body tissues and have powerful anti-cancer effects.

So it makes sense to tuck into plenty of vegetables. Here are some easy recipes.

A special word on potatoes. Potatoes are a great food. They are excellent sources of vitamins, fibre and minerals, taste good and fill you up. Contrary to old-fashioned ideas, spuds won't make you fat because, by themselves, they contain no fat. Unfortunately, potatoes are usually served with some type of fat. For example, chips are cooked in oil (or dripping, in the case of commercially-prepared chips), roast potatoes soak up meat fat, mashed potatoes have butter or margarine, jacket potatoes are topped with sour cream. It's the fat that so often accompanies potatoes that causes weight problems, not the potatoes themselves. This chapter shows you some delicious easy ways to cook potatoes—and other vegetables—without drowning them in fat.

Herb stuffed spuds
Spinach stuffed spuds
Corn and turkey ham stuffed spuds
Sun-dried tomato and mushroom stuffed spuds
Chilli and coriander stuffed spuds
Crispy potato pancakes
Spanish potato omelette
Fluffy potato souffles
Potato and celery cake
Hot potato salad
Baked stuffed eggplant
Zucchini stir-fry
Barbecued leeks
Barbecued mushrooms
Cauliflower with rich tomato sauce
Beans and corn
Sesame snow peas and beans
Spicy broccoli
Carrots and mushrooms with lemon dressing
Curried vegetables

Herb stuffed spuds

Desiree or Pontiac potatoes are especially good for baking and stuffing.

    4 medium to large potatoes, scrubbed
    ½ cup low-fat smooth ricotta cheese
    2 teaspoons Dijon mustard
    ½ cup chopped fresh basil
    1 tablespoon chopped mint
    freshly ground pepper

1. Bake potatoes on oven shelf at 180°C for about 1¼ hours, or until tender when pierced with a skewer. Alternatively, cook potatoes on High in microwave for 12 to 15 minutes. Remove from oven, cut a lid from each potato and scoop out flesh, taking care to leave enough potato next to the skin to form a shell.
2. Mash potato with ricotta, mustard, basil, mint and pepper. Pile mashed potato back into potato shells and bake in a moderate oven for 15 minutes (or microwave on High for 4 to 5 minutes).

Serves 4
Fat per serve: 2 grams

Spinach stuffed spuds

Even if you're not fond of spinach, it tastes great when used as a stuffing for potatoes. Try to find some English spinach which has a milder flavour than silverbeet.

4 medium to large potatoes, scrubbed
½ bunch English spinach
½ cup low-fat natural yoghurt
pinch nutmeg
2 tablespoons chopped shallots
1 tablespoon lemon juice

1. Bake potatoes on oven shelf at 180°C for about 1¼ hours, or until tender when pierced with a skewer. Alternatively, cook potatoes on High in microwave for 12 to 15 minutes. Remove from oven, cut a lid from each potato and scoop out flesh, taking care to leave enough potato next to the skin to form a shell.
2. While potatoes are baking, wash and steam spinach until just wilted. Cool and then squeeze spinach tightly to remove as much water as possible. Chop finely.
3. Combine potato flesh with spinach, yoghurt, nutmeg, shallots and lemon juice. Pile back into potato shells and bake in a moderate oven for 15 minutes (or microwave on High for 4 to 5 minutes).

Serves 4
Fat per serve: 0

Corn and turkey ham stuffed spuds

Turkey ham (sometimes called 'turkey hamwich') is low in fat but adds a good, almost bacon-like flavour. It goes well in these hearty spuds.

4 large potatoes, scrubbed
1 tablespoon chopped mint
freshly ground pepper
½ cup low-fat natural yoghurt
1 cup drained corn kernels
1 cup chopped turkey ham

1. Bake potatoes on oven shelf at 180°C for about 1¼ hours, or until tender when pierced with a skewer. Alternatively, cook potatoes on High in microwave for 12 to 15 minutes. Remove from oven, cut a lid from each potato and scoop out flesh, taking care to leave enough potato next to the skin to form a shell.

2. Mash potato flesh, adding mint, pepper and yoghurt. Fold in corn kernels and turkey ham. Pile back into potato shells and bake in a moderate oven for 15 minutes (or microwave on High for 4 to 5 minutes).

Serves 4
Fat per serve: 2 grams

Sun-dried tomato and mushroom stuffed spuds

Some sun-dried tomatoes are packed in oil. Drain them well before using.

4 medium to large potatoes, scrubbed
½ cup low-fat cottage cheese
freshly ground pepper
2 tablespoons chopped basil
2 tablespoons sun-dried tomatoes, cut into strips
1 cup finely chopped mushrooms

1. Bake potatoes on oven shelf at 180°C for about 1¼ hours, or until tender when pierced with a skewer. Alternatively, cook potatoes on High in microwave for 12 to 15 minutes. Remove from oven, cut a lid from each potato and scoop out flesh, taking care to leave enough potato next to the skin to form a shell.
2. Mash potato flesh with cottage cheese, pepper and basil. Mix in sun-dried tomatoes and mushrooms and pile back into potato shells. Bake in a moderate oven for 15 minutes (or microwave on High for 4 to 5 minutes).

Serves 4
Fat per serve: 2 grams (assuming there is a little residual oil on tomatoes)

Chilli and coriander stuffed spuds

These potatoes are wonderful with grilled chicken or barbecued fish and salad.

    4 medium potatoes, scrubbed
    1 bunch coriander
    ½ cup low-fat yoghurt
    2 small chillies, seeded and chopped*

    * take care not to rub eyes when handling chilli as
      their naturally-occurring chemicals can damage the
      delicate tissues in the eye

1. Bake potatoes on oven shelf at 180°C for about 1¼ hours, or until tender when pierced with a skewer. Alternatively, cook potatoes on High in microwave for 12 to 15 minutes. Remove from oven, cut a lid from each potato and scoop out flesh, taking care to leave enough potato next to the skin to form a shell.
2. Remove roots from coriander and chop leaves and stems finely.
3. Mash potato flesh with yoghurt, chilli and coriander and pile back into potato shells. Bake in a moderate oven for 15 minutes (or microwave on High for 4 to 5 minutes).

Serves 4
Fat per serve: 0

Crispy potato pancakes

Cooked until they're crisp and golden, these potato pancakes are better for you than chips. Try to use a heavy-based non-stick pan and keep the heat low to prevent them burning. Top with a little chilli, if you like them hot.

approximately 750 g potatoes, peeled*
1 medium onion
¼ cup self-raising flour
1 teaspoon dried oregano or marjoram leaves
1 egg
1 extra egg white
freshly ground pepper
2 teaspoons olive oil

* if using new scrubbed potatoes, don't bother to peel them

1. Grate potatoes and onion using a coarse grater or food processor. Using your hands, squeeze potatoes to extract as much moisture as possible.
2. Add flour, oregano, egg and extra egg white, and pepper to potato. Mix well, adding a little more flour if mixture seems to be too wet. (This depends on how much water you have been able to squeeze from the potatoes.)
3. Brush half a teaspoon of olive oil over a heavy-based hot pan. Add tablespoons of potato mixture to the hot pan, turn heat down and cook over a gentle heat for 3 to 4 minutes on each side. Remove first batch of pancakes and keep warm while using remaining mixture.

Makes about 8 and serves 4
Fat per serve: 4 grams

Spanish potato omelette

A true Spanish omelette does not contain tomatoes or capsicum but is made from potatoes, onions and eggs. This version is low in fat and is equally delicious served hot with a main meal or left to have cold for the next day's lunch.

750 g potatoes, peeled and sliced thinly*
2 large onions, sliced thinly*
4 eggs
2 egg whites
½ teaspoon ground black pepper
2 teaspoons olive oil, preferably extra virgin

* a food processor makes this easy

1. Steam or microwave potato and onion slices until almost tender.
2. Heat a heavy-based pan, add oil. Arrange potato and onion slices in layers in pan.
3. Beat eggs, extra egg whites and pepper. Pour this mixture over potato in pan and cook on a low heat for 10 to 12 minutes or until egg is almost set. Place pan under griller to finish cooking top. If serving cold, refrigerate until required.

---

*Serves 4 to 6
Fat per serve: 6 to 8 grams (to
reduce fat, use a non-stick pan and
halve or omit olive oil)*

Fluffy potato souffles

Easy to make and always popular. A great dish for lovers of mashed potato.

750 g potatoes
½ cup sliced green shallots
freshly ground pepper
1 tablespoon chopped chives
¼ cup low-fat milk
1 egg yolk, beaten
2 egg whites
1 tablespoon finely grated Parmesan cheese

1. Steam or microwave potatoes until tender. Peel and mash, adding shallots, pepper, chives, milk and egg yolk.
2. Beat egg whites until stiff. Fold a little of the egg whites into the potato mixture and mix lightly, then gently fold in remaining egg white. Do not beat or mix too hard or the egg whites will lose their fluffiness.
3. Divide mixture between 4 medium or 6 small souffle dishes. Sprinkle top with Parmesan and bake in a moderate oven for about 20 minutes, or until well risen and brown. Serve at once.

Serves 4 to 6
Fat per serve: 2 grams

Potato and celery cake

This is another recipe that tastes good when it's cold. Take some to work with a salad and buy a fresh roll to go with it.

750 g potatoes, peeled
1 medium onion, grated
1 cup finely sliced celery
2 eggs
1 tablespoon lemon juice
1 cup instant skim milk powder
1 tablespoon chopped fresh rosemary (or use
   1 teaspoon dried)
1 teaspoon olive oil
1 slice wholemeal bread, made into breadcrumbs
1 tablespoon finely grated Parmesan cheese

1. Grate potatoes and onion (use a food processor). Using your hands, squeeze as much moisture from potato mixture as possible.
2. Combine potato and onion with celery. Toss well together.
3. Beat eggs and lemon juice. Combine eggs with potato mixture, and add skim milk powder and rosemary, mixing well.
4. Brush oil over a non-stick cake tin and press potato cake into tin. Sprinkle with breadcrumbs and Parmesan cheese and bake in a moderate oven for 40 minutes. Serve cut into wedges.

Serves 4 to 6
Fat per serve: 4 to 6 grams

Hot potato salad

Good on a cold day, either on its own or as an accompaniment to the main meal.

600 g small new potatoes
2 teaspoons olive oil
1 medium onion, chopped finely
1 clove garlic, crushed
400 g can tomatoes, chopped roughly
2 tablespoons chopped parsley

1. If potatoes are not very small, cut in halves. Do not peel. Steam or microwave potatoes until tender.
2. While potatoes are cooking, heat oil and gently cook onion and garlic for 3 to 4 minutes, without browning. Add tomatoes, bring to the boil and simmer, uncovered, for about 10 to 15 minutes.
3. Pour tomato mixture over hot potatoes and top with chopped parsley.

Serves 4
Fat per serve: 3 grams

Baked stuffed eggplant

You could also use this stuffing in small pumpkins, capsicums, tomatoes or, if you have the patience to assemble them, in hollowed-out zucchini.

> 2 eggplants, each about 250–300 g
> 2 teaspoons olive oil
> 1 small onion, chopped finely
> 1 teaspoon dried basil leaves
> ½ cup chopped turkey ham or turkey salami (low fat)
> 1 cup cooked brown rice
> 1 egg
> ½ cup chopped parsley
> 1 tablespoon Parmesan cheese

1. Pierce eggplants with a skewer in several places and bake on the shelf of a moderate oven for 25 minutes, or cook, uncovered, in microwave on High for 10 minutes. Remove from oven, cool a little, cut in halves and carefully scoop out the middle. Chop this finely.
2. Heat oil and gently cook onion and basil for 2 to 3 minutes.
3. Add chopped eggplant flesh, turkey ham, rice, egg and parsley. Mix well and pile back into eggplant shells. Sprinkle with Parmesan and bake in a moderate oven for 20 minutes or microwave on High for 8–10 minutes.

Serves 4
Fat per serve: 6 grams

Zucchini stir-fry

Turn yourself into a popular cook with this easy recipe. Great to feed kids who say they don't like vegetables.

400 g zucchini
250 g carrots
250 g celeriac (or use 2 sticks sliced celery)
1 tablespoon sesame oil
1 tablespoon chopped chives

1. Grate vegetables, using a coarse grater. Mix well together.
2. Heat oil in a heavy-based non-stick frying pan. Add vegetables and stir-fry for about 2 to 3 minutes. Add chives, toss well and serve at once.

Serves 4
Fat per serve: 5 grams

Barbecued leeks

*Many vegetables taste good wrapped in foil and barbe-
cued. Leeks are especially delicious—and very easy to
prepare.*

>   2 large leeks
>   1 teaspoon olive oil
>   2 cloves garlic, crushed
>   1 tablespoon chopped fresh oregano (or thyme)

1. Trim coarse outer leaves of leeks, especially near
   the top, but do not remove all the green. Wash
   leeks well, separating green part to remove dirt.
   Cut each leek in half crosswise and then cut each
   half again lengthwise.
2. Cut two pieces of foil a little larger than the leeks.
   Brush each piece of foil with olive oil and sprinkle
   the centre with garlic and oregano. Place 4 pieces
   of leek on top of garlic and oregano on each piece
   of foil and wrap up to form a parcel. Barbecue for
   20 minutes. Delicious with any barbecued meats,
   fish or chicken.

Serves 4
Fat per serve: 1 gram

Barbecued mushrooms

There is no better way to discover the wonderful flavour of mushrooms than this.

8 large flat mushrooms, or 16 smaller button
   mushrooms
1 teaspoon olive oil
1 teaspoon finely grated lemon rind
2 tablespoons chopped parsley

Cut 4 pieces of foil, each large enough to hold 2 flat mushrooms. Brush foil with olive oil and sprinkle centre with lemon rind and parsley. Place mushrooms on top of parsley, fold up parcels and barbecue for 15 minutes.

Serves 4
Fat per serve: 1 gram

Cauliflower with rich tomato sauce

Cauliflower has traditionally been served with parsley sauce. This rich tomato sauce has much more flavour. It is also delicious served with zucchini or steamed leeks.

1 small cauliflower, or half a larger one
2 teaspoons olive oil
1 medium onion, finely chopped
1 clove garlic, crushed
1 teaspoon chopped chilli
1 slice wholemeal bread
400 g fresh tomatoes, cored and chopped roughly
1 teaspoon paprika
2 tablespoons red wine vinegar
½ teaspoon black pepper

1. Cut cauliflower into individual pieces and steam for 4 to 5 minutes or microwave in a covered container on High for 2 minutes. Do not overcook cauliflower—it should be barely tender. Place cauliflower in shallow dish.
2. Heat oil in saucepan and cook onion, garlic and chilli over a gentle heat for 3 to 4 minutes.
3. Using a blender or food processor, make bread into crumbs. Add to blender or processor the onion mixture, tomatoes, paprika, vinegar and pepper. Blend to form a paste. Pour over cauliflower and bake in a moderate oven for 10 minutes or heat in microwave on High for 5 to 6 minutes, or until piping hot.

Serves 4
Fat per serve: 3 grams

Beans and corn

This recipe tells you how to cook beans from scratch. If you prefer, simply open a 680 g can of beans, drain them and proceed from step 2.

1 cup (200 g) red kidney beans
1 teaspoon dried thyme
water
250 g frozen corn kernels or 440 g can corn
   kernels, drained
1 teaspoon chopped chilli (optional)
½ cup chopped parsley

1. Place beans in a large saucepan and cover with water. Leave to soak overnight. Pour off soaking water and replace with fresh water. Add thyme. Bring to the boil, cover and simmer for about 1¼ hours, or until beans are just tender. Drain.
2. Combine beans, corn and chilli in a saucepan and stir over medium heat until hot. Add parsley.

Serves 6
Fat per serve: 1 gram

Sesame snow peas and beans

Snow peas are always popular. Combined with green beans and flavoured with sesame, they taste terrific.

    2 teaspoons sesame seeds
    400 g green beans
    200 g snow peas
    1 teaspoon sesame oil
    1 clove garlic, crushed

1. Toast sesame seeds in a dry frying pan over a gentle heat, shaking frequently until seeds turn golden brown (take care not to burn them). Set aside.
2. Cut off ends of beans and snow peas. Steam for no more than 3 minutes or microwave for 2 minutes.
3. Heat sesame oil and gently saute garlic for a minute or so. Add beans and peas and toss well together until hot. Sprinkle with reserved sesame seeds.

Serves 4
Fat per serve: 2 grams

Spicy broccoli

Here's a simple way to add flavour to broccoli. To save time, you can buy chopped chilli and ginger in jars.

1 tablespoon peanut or vegetable oil
2 medium onions, sliced
2 cloves garlic
2 teaspoons chopped ginger
1 teaspoon chopped chilli
2 teaspoons coriander seeds
1 teaspoon cumin seeds
500 g broccoli, trimmed and cut into small pieces
½ cup water

1. Heat oil in large pan and cook onions, garlic, ginger, chilli, coriander and cumin seeds over a low heat, covered, for about 10 minutes. Stir occasionally.
2. Add broccoli and water, cover and cook for about 5 minutes, or until broccoli is just tender.

Serves 4
Fat per serve: 5 grams

Carrots and mushrooms with lemon dressing

By combining vegetables and adding a touch of dressing you make them more interesting.

  1 teaspoon olive oil
  1 small onion, sliced
  2 large carrots, cut into thin slices
  ½ cup chicken stock
  250 g mushrooms, sliced
  1 tablespoon lemon juice
  1 tablespoon chopped mint

1. Heat oil in saucepan, add onion, cover and cook over a gentle heat for 2 minutes. Add carrots and stock, bring to the boil, cover and simmer for 5 minutes.
2. Add mushrooms and continue cooking with the lid off for a further 3 minutes, stirring occasionally. Add lemon juice and mint, toss well and serve, pouring any remaining juice over vegetables.

Serves 4
Fat per serve: 1 gram

Curried vegetables

Use any vegetables you have for this simple dish. If you do not have any chick pea flour you can omit it, but take care not to boil the yoghurt or it will curdle.

1 teaspoon cumin seeds, preferably black cumin if you can find them
1 teaspoon black mustard seeds
1 teaspoon peanut or vegetable oil
1 teaspoon chopped chilli
2 teaspoons chopped ginger
1 clove garlic, crushed
1 tablespoon ground coriander
1 teaspoon turmeric
6 cups vegetables (green beans, carrot, pumpkin, broccoli, cauliflower, eggplant, capsicum, okra)
½ cup water
200 g carton low-fat natural yoghurt
1 teaspoon chick pea flour*
½ cup chopped fresh coriander

* available from some health food shops or Asian greengrocers

1. In a dry pan with a lid, heat cumin and mustard seeds until they pop.
2. Add oil, chilli, ginger, garlic, ground coriander and turmeric and cook over a gentle heat for 2 to 3 minutes.
3. Add vegetables and water, cover and simmer for about 10 minutes.
4. Blend yoghurt and pea flour and stir into vegetable mixture. Add fresh coriander and serve at once.

Serves 4
Fat per serve: 1 gram

Desserts

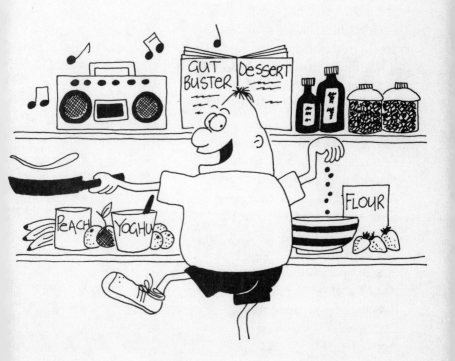

There's no escaping the fact that the ideal dessert is fresh
fruit. There's also no escaping the fact that most of us
occasionally want something other than fresh fruit for dessert.

Many desserts take a lot of preparation time. I have
assumed that anyone reading this book wants easy, fast
recipes—so that's what I have included.

This chapter does not attempt to give you chocolate
puddings without chocolate, or cakes without sugar or fat.
Some dishes just *can't* be made without using the real
ingredients. But there are some delicious low-fat desserts
that you can whip up when the urge takes you. Try some.

Strawberries with a difference
Dried fruit salad
Fresh fruit salads
    Summer fresh fruit salad
    Stone fresh fruit salad
    Summer berry salad
    Autumn fruit salad
Spicy fruits with yoghurt
Peaches poached in white wine
Mango and pawpaw freeze
Jellied berries and cherries
Rhubarb and apple crumble
Orange crepes
Melon sorbet
Peachy pancakes
Baked stuffed apples
Peach sponge pudding
Lemon sauce pudding
Apricot loaf
Teatime date cake
Ricotta whip

Strawberries with a difference

*If you've never tasted strawberries with balsamic vinegar,
try them soon. They're delicious.*

    2 punnets fresh strawberries
    1 tablespoon icing sugar
    2 tablespoons balsamic vinegar*

    * available from delicatessens

Hull strawberries and place in serving dishes. Sprinkle
with icing sugar and toss gently. Sprinkle with balsamic
vinegar.

Serves 4
Fat per serve: 0

Dried fruit salad

An ideal fruit salad to make in winter.

   1 cup water
   1 cinnamon stick
   6 cloves
   4 cardamom pods
   250 g dried fruits (apples, apricots, peaches,
      nectarines, prunes)
   1 cup fruit juice

Heat water with cinnamon stick, cloves and cardamom
pods. Add juice and dried fruits, bring to the boil, cover
and simmer for 15 minutes. Leave to cool in saucepan.
Chill well. Remove cinnamon stick, cloves and cardamom pods before serving.

Serves 4
Fat per serve: 0

Fresh fruit salads

The secret to a good fruit salad is using fruits in season. Always try to include at least one fragrant fruit too—for example, passionfruit, rockmelon, nectarines, mango. You can prevent fruits such as bananas going brown when their cut surfaces are exposed to oxygen by brushing them with lemon juice or preparing them just before you're ready to eat them.

Summer fresh fruit salad

½ an average-sized rockmelon, peeled and diced
½ an average-sized pineapple, peeled and diced
250 g sultana grapes
1 punnet strawberries
flesh of 6 passionfruit
2 bananas, peeled and sliced
2 kiwi fruit, peeled and sliced
2 tablespoons fresh orange juice

Combine all fruits except banana. Sprinkle with orange juice and chill for one hour. Just before serving, add banana.

Serves 4 to 6
Fat per serve: 0

Stone fresh fruit salad

2 mangoes
4 peaches
12 apricots
4 blood plums
250 g cherries

Peel all fruits and cut flesh into chunks. Toss well
together. Chill well before serving. Serve in a glass bowl
set within a larger glass bowl filled with ice. This keeps
the fruits in beautiful condition.

Serves 4
Fat per serve: 0

Summer berry salad

> 250 g frozen raspberries
> 2 tablespoons orange juice
> 1 tablespoon castor sugar (or use sugar substitute)
> 1 punnet strawberries, hulls removed
> 1 punnet blueberries
> 1 punnet raspberries

1. Thaw frozen raspberries and combine with orange
   juice and sugar (or substitute). Blend until smooth.
   (If you like a really smooth effect, this sauce may
   be sieved as well.)
2. Combine strawberries, blueberries and raspberries
   and toss gently together. Place into individual serving dishes. Pour some of the raspberry sauce over
   the top of the fruit.

Serves 4 to 6
Fat per serve: 0

Autumn fruit salad

> 1 tablespoon flaked almonds
> 2 oranges
> 2 pears

2 apples
¼ cup lemon juice
1 tablespoon icing sugar
2 kiwi fruit, peeled and quartered

1. Toast almonds in a dry frying pan over a low heat, shaking frequently, until golden brown. Take care they do not burn. Set aside to cool.
2. Peel oranges, making sure there is no pith remaining. Cut into slices.
3. Core and peel pears and core apples. Cut both into dice and toss with orange slices and lemon juice. Sprinkle with icing sugar.
4. To serve, place one-quarter of the fruits into each plate and top with two kiwi fruit quarters and one quarter of the almonds.

Serves 4
Fat per serve: 2 grams

Spicy fruits with yoghurt

It takes only a few minutes to mix this dessert but the flavour improves if you can make it an hour before you need it and leave it in the fridge.

1 punnet blueberries (or strawberries)
1 orange, peeled and sliced
1 grapefruit, peeled, pith removed and cut into segments
2 bananas, peeled and sliced
2 cups seedless green grapes*
500 g low-fat natural yoghurt
1 teaspoon cinnamon
½ teaspoon ground cardamom
pinch nutmeg

* if grapes are out of season, use a can of pie-pack peaches instead

1. Place all fruits into a bowl.
2. Stir spices into yoghurt, pour over fruit and toss gently together. Allow to stand for an hour, if possible, to allow flavours to mingle.

Serves 4
Fat per serve: 0

Peaches poached in white wine

Make this dessert when fresh peaches are in season. It is particularly good with white peaches.

4 fresh peaches
1 cup white wine
1 tablespoon honey
1 piece of cinnamon stick
grated rind of 1 lemon

1. Skin peaches by placing them in a bowl or saucepan and pouring boiling water over them. Leave for 1 minute then drain. Skin will peel off easily.
2. Place whole peaches in a saucepan with remaining ingredients. Bring to the boil, cover and simmer for 5 minutes. Turn heat off and leave until cold. Place peaches into a clean dish and strain liquid over them. Chill well before serving with low-fat fromage frais.

Serves 4
Fat per serve: 0

Mango and pawpaw freeze

This is not the same as having a rich ice-cream. But it is refreshingly delicious. You can use an artificial sweetener instead of the sugar if you want to save on kilojoules.

2 mangoes, peeled
1 small pawpaw, peeled and seeded
2 tablespoons lime juice
½ cup sugar
500 g low-fat natural yoghurt
1 tablespoon gelatine
½ cup orange juice

1. Cut off mango flesh and place in blender or food processor with diced pawpaw, lime juice and sugar. Blend well. Add yoghurt and stir to combine.
2. Mix gelatine and orange juice and dissolve by heating gently or microwaving for about 15 seconds. Add to mango mixture. Pour into an ice-cream churn and follow manufacturer's instructions, or pour into a cake tin and freeze until almost solid. Remove from freezer and beat in an electric mixer until smooth. Re-freeze until solid.

Serves 4
Fat per serve: 0

Jellied berries and cherries

Great on a really hot day but it needs to be made several hours before you want to eat it. Taste the juices and fruits. If they aren't sweet enough, you may want to add some artificial sweetener to taste.

1 punnet strawberries
1 punnet blueberries
500 g fresh cherries
2 tablespoons gelatine
1 cup hot water
2 cups grape juice

1. Place berries and cherries into a ring tin or a glass dish.
2. Dissolve gelatine in hot water. Add grape juice. Pour over berries and refrigerate until set.

Serves 4
Fat per serve: 0

Rhubarb and apple crumble

Most crumbles have a high fat content because the butter they contain holds them together. This recipe is for a true crumble. Without much fat, it doesn't stick together but crumbles. Make it in individual dishes for the best results. It tastes great.

1 bunch rhubarb, cut into 3 cm lengths
1 tablespoon orange juice
400 g can pie-pack apples
2 teaspoons cinnamon
1 tablespoon sunflower seeds
2 tablespoons fat-reduced butter
1/3 cup dark brown sugar
1 cup rolled oats
1/2 cup processed bran cereal

1. Place rhubarb and orange juice into a saucepan, cover and cook over a gentle heat for about 5–8 minutes, or until rhubarb is just cooked. Add apples and 1 teaspoon of cinnamon and place in 6 individual souffle-style dishes (or use one larger casserole dish).

2. Place sunflower seeds in a dry frying pan and heat gently, shaking often, until seeds are golden brown (take care they do not burn). Set aside.

3. Combine fat-reduced butter, sugar, remaining cinnamon, oats and bran cereal and mix well. Add sunflower seeds. Tip mixture on top of rhubarb and apple and press down gently. Bake in a moderate oven for 30 minutes. Serve hot with low-fat fromage frais or low-fat ice-cream.

Serves 6
Fat per serve: 6 grams

Orange crepes

It's good fun to make crepes. Don't toss them too much or they will be leathery.

1 cup flour
1 cup low-fat milk
3 eggs
light olive oil

Orange sauce
3 oranges
¾ cup orange juice
1 teaspoon cornflour
1 tablespoon finely grated orange rind
2 tablespoons orange liqueur
1 cup low kilojoule orange marmalade

1. In blender combine flour, milk and eggs. Leave to stand for at least 30 minutes.
2. Peel oranges, taking care to remove all pith. Slice.
3. Combine 2 tablespoons orange juice with cornflour, stirring until smooth. Heat remaining juice with orange rind and bring to the boil. Add cornflour mixture and stir until slightly thickened. Add liqueur and orange slices and set aside.
4. Heat a non-stick pan and brush with light olive oil. Pour in about 2 tablespoons of the crepe mixture, swirl and cook until lightly brown. Turn and cook other side. Stack crepes until you have used all the mixture.
5. Spoon a good teaspoon of low kilojoule marmalade onto each crepe. Fold in quarters.
6. Heat orange sauce in a frying pan, add crepes and gently move in the sauce until crepes are warm.

Serves 4 to 6
Fat per serve: 4 to 6 grams

Melon sorbet

Nothing beats a cooling sorbet on a hot day. I like to make melon sorbets from watermelon, rockmelon and honeydew melon and serve a scoop of each.

    2 cups rockmelon flesh
    2 cups honeydew melon flesh
    2 or 3 mint leaves
    2 cups watermelon flesh
    4 egg whites
    6 tablespoons sugar

1. Puree rockmelon and pour into a bowl.
2. Puree honeydew and mint and pour into a bowl.
3. Puree watermelon and pour into a bowl.
4. In a clean, dry bowl, beat egg whites until stiff, adding sugar gradually and continuing to beat until the mixture looks like a shiny meringue.
5. Place one-third of the egg white mixture on top of each of the three melon purees and fold in carefully until just combined. Place into cake tins and freeze until almost solid. Remove from freezer, beat each one well and return to freezer until solid.

Serves 6
Fat per serve: 0

Peachy pancakes

Pancakes are not as sinful as many people imagine. Made the low-fat way, you hardly notice any difference from regular pancakes. But please serve them with fruit, ricotta whip (see page 140), frozen Vitari or a low-fat fromage frais. There's no way cream fits into a gut-buster program.

¾ cup wholemeal self-raising flour
¾ cup plain flour
¼ teaspoon baking powder
¾ cup low-fat milk
1 tablespoon honey
2 eggs
vegetable oil

Filling
400 g can peaches (without added sugar)
½ teaspoon cinnamon
1 tablespoon cornflour
1 tablespoon lemon juice

1. In blender or food processor, combine flours, baking powder, milk and honey. Blend until smooth and allow to stand for 30 minutes (or longer).
2. To prepare filling: reserve 2 tablespoons peach juice and blend with cornflour.
3. Heat peaches and the remaining juice with cinnamon. Add cornflour mixture and lemon juice, stirring constantly until mixture thickens. Set aside.
4. To make pancakes: heat a heavy-based non-stick frying pan. Brush with a little vegetable oil and pour in about 3 tablespoons of mixture. Cook until bubbles appear, turn and cook other side until brown. Stack cooked pancakes.

5. Place a spoonful of filling on one pancake, roll up and place in a shallow ovenproof dish. Continue until all pancakes and filling have been used. Reheat in microwave, covered with plastic film, for 6 to 8 minutes or cover with foil and reheat in a moderate oven (180°C) for 15 minutes. Serve any remaining filling beside pancakes.

Serves 4 to 6
Fat per serve: 2 to 3 grams

Baked stuffed apples

One of the easiest desserts to make, and very fast if you have a microwave oven. Use any dried fruit you like to stuff the centre of baked apples.

4 medium Granny Smith apples
4 dried apricot halves
1 tablespoon raisins
¾ cup apple juice

1. Core apples, using an apple corer or a sharp knife. Run knife around centre of apple, cutting through the skin with a shallow cut (this stops the apples bursting when they are baked).
2. Stuff a dried apricot and a few raisins into the centre of each apple. Place in a casserole dish just large enough to hold all the apples. Pour apple juice over apples and bake in a moderate oven for 30 minutes, or cover loosely with plastic wrap and microwave on High for about 5 minutes, or until apples are just tender.

Serves 4
Fat per serve: 0

Peach sponge pudding

This dessert is low in fat but the sugar does increase the kilojoules. Substitute Slenda artificial sweetener if you like.

> 800 g pie-pack peaches
> 1 teaspoon cinnamon
> 2 eggs
> ⅓ cup sugar
> 1 tablespoon concentrated orange juice
> ½ cup self-raising flour
> 1 tablespoon cornflour

1. Combine peaches and cinnamon and spread over the base of a small casserole dish (about 1.5 L capacity).
2. Beat eggs and sugar until thick and creamy. Add orange juice. Gently fold in sifted flours and mix lightly until just combined. Pour over peaches and bake in a moderate oven for 30 minutes.

Serves 4
Fat per serve: 3 grams

Lemon sauce pudding

A light sponge-type pudding with its own sauce. Good for a cold winter evening. Also delicious with grapefruit or orange replacing the lemon.

½ cup water
½ cup lemon juice
½ cup sugar
2 tablespoons flour
2 eggs, separated
½ cup skim milk powder

1. Into blender place water, lemon juice, half the sugar, flour, egg yolks and skim milk powder. Blend until smooth.
2. Beat egg whites until stiff, adding remaining sugar. Gently fold egg whites into lemon mixture. Pour into an ovenproof dish. Place in a larger container, such as a baking dish, containing water to come halfway up the sides. Bake in a moderate oven for 35 to 40 minutes, or until set. Serve hot.

Serves 4
Fat per serve: 3 grams

Apricot loaf

You can whip this loaf up with little effort. It keeps well and tastes good.

    200 g dried apricots
    1 cup orange juice
    1 egg, beaten
    1 cup wholemeal self-raising flour
    ½ cup self-raising flour
    1 teaspoon cinnamon
    ½ teaspoon allspice

1. Place apricots and orange juice into a saucepan, bring to the boil, cover and simmer for 2 minutes. Turn off heat and leave until cool.
2. Add to apricots the beaten egg, sifted flours and spices. Mix well. Spoon mixture into a non-stick loaf tin lined with baking paper. Bake in a moderate oven for 40 minutes, or until a skewer inserted into the centre comes out clean.

Makes 16 slices
Fat per slice: 0.5 gram

Teatime date cake

This loaf is not too sweet. Serve it thinly sliced, on its own or spread with a little fat-reduced butter.

2 cups cold black tea
1 cup seeded chopped dates
1 teaspoon bi-carb soda
1 teaspoon cinnamon
2 teaspoons finely grated lemon rind
2 tablespoons lemon juice
1½ cups wholemeal self-raising flour
1 tablespoon poppy seeds

1. Place in a saucepan the tea, dates, carb-soda, cinnamon and lemon rind. Bring to the boil, cover and simmer for 5 minutes. Add lemon juice and leave to cool.
2. Sift flour and add date mixture. Mix well and pour into a non-stick loaf tin, lined with baking paper. Sprinkle poppy seeds on top, pressing them lightly into mixture with the back of a spoon. Bake in a moderate oven for 40 minutes, or until a skewer inserted into the centre comes out clean.

Makes 16 slices
Fat per slice: 0.5 gram

Ricotta whip

A light topping that can be used as a substitute for cream.

½ cup dried apricots
½ cup orange juice
1 cup smooth ricotta cheese

1. Combine apricots and orange juice and cook over a gentle heat until apricots are pulpy (time will vary according to dryness of apricots). Blend until smooth and set aside until cool.
2. Add ricotta to blender and puree until smooth.

Serves 6
Fat per serve: 3 grams

Index